Pediatric Neurology for the House Officer

Third Edition

D0939945

Pediatric Neurology for the House Officer

Third Edition

Howard L. Weiner, M.D.

Center for Neurological Diseases
Brigham and Women's Hospital
Boston, Massachusetts

David K. Urion, M.D.

Department of Neurology
The Children's Hospital
Boston, Massachusetts

Lawrence P. Levitt, M.D.

Division of Neurology
Allentown Hospital
Allentown and Sacred Heart Hospital Center
Allentown, Pennsylvania

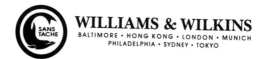

WILLIAMS & WILKINS
BALTIMORE · HONG KONG · LONDON · MUNICH
PHILADELPHIA · SYDNEY · TOKYO

Editor: Michael G. Fisher
Associate Editor: Carol Eckhart
Copy Editor: Deborah Tourtlotte
Design: Bob Och
Illustration Planning: Raymond Lowman
Production: Charles E. Zeller
Cover Design: Dan Pfisterer

Copyright © 1988
Williams & Wilkins
428 East Preston Street
Baltimore, MD 21202, USA

Accurate indications, adverse reactions, and dosage schedules for drugs are provided in this book, but it is possible that they may change. The reader is urged to review the package information data of the manufacturers of the medications mentioned.

Printed in the United States of America

Second Edition 1982

Library of Congress Cataloging in Publication Data

Weiner, Howard L.
  Pediatric neurology for the house officer / Howard L. Weiner.
David K. Urion, Lawrence P. Levitt.—3rd ed.
    p.   cm.
  Includes bibliographies and index.
  ISBN 0-683-08904-8
  1. Pediatric neurology—Handbooks, manuals, etc. I. Urion, David K. II. Levitt,
Lawrence P. III. Title
RJ486.W35   1988
618.92'8—dc19   88-12069
                                                                      CIP

10   9   8   7   6   5

Dedication

To: Michael J. Bresnan, exemplary physician, teacher, and friend.

Foreword

This third edition of <u>Pediatric Neurology for the</u>
<u>House Officer</u> represents the collaboration of Howard
Weiner, David Urion, and Lawrence Levitt. Dr. Urion takes
over the late Dr. Michael Bresnan, Co-Author of the first
two editions of this book. Dr. Bresnan's premature death
leaves a gap in the lives of his colleagues; much of his
approach to the child with suspected neurologic disease
continues to reverberate throughout this text.

It is more than unsettling to realize that a
second generation of one's students has taken over the
first in the editing of the text. More than a sign of
advancing age, it also represents the institution of
certain things you have said over the years as an oral
tradition now recorded in print. Our colleagues on the
staff will also recognize some of their favorite
teachings. Full credit goes to the authors for putting it
altogether, adding points from their own experience in
literature, and making a choice amongst the occasional
contraversial views among us.

As I pointed out in the foreword to the first
edition of this book, neurology is still the most
consulted service in the hospital. It is our business,
and we like it. It also indicates something of the unease
of our pediatric colleagues about neurologic problems.
This manual continues to provide straight answers to the
frequent questions that arise. Moreover, it stimulates
further questions about clinical problems and I hope will
continue to stimulate general interest in the nervous
system among its pediatric readers.

I am certain that the third edition of <u>Pediatric Neurology for the House Officer</u> will continue to meet the practical needs of physicians in recognizing and treating neurologic diseases in the child.

Charles F. Barlow, M.D.
Bronson Crothers Professor
 of Neurology
Harvard Medical School

About the Authors

Howard L. Weiner, M.D., is Physician in Medicine
(Neurology) at the Brigham and Women's Hospital and Robert
L. Kroc Associate Professor of Neurologic Diseases at
Harvard Medical School. He attended Dartmouth College and
the University of Colorado Medical School; he then
interned at Chaim Sheba Hospital, Tel Hashomer, Israel,
and served as a medical resident at the Beth Israel
Hospital, Boston. Dr. Weiner is Director of the Multiple
Sclerosis Clinical and Research Unit and Co-Director of
the Center for Neurologic Diseases at the Brighamm and
Women's Hospital.

David K. Urion, M.D., is Director of Learning Disabilities
and Behavioral Neurology at Children's Hospital and
Assistant Professor of Neurology at Harvard Medical
School. He graduated from the Stanford University School
of Medicine; he interned at Peter Bent Brigham Hospital,
was a Pediatric Resident at Children's Hospital, and
trained in Neurology in the Longwood Area Neurology
Training Program. His main interests are in clinical
pediatric neurology and learning disorders.

Lawrence P. Levitt, M.D., is Senior Consultant in
Neurology at the Allentown Hospital-Lehigh Valley Hospital
Center in Allentown, Pennsylvania. He is Clinical
Professor of Neurology at Hahnemann University, and
Clinical Associate Professor of Neurology at Temple
University School of Medicine. A graduate of Queens
College, he then attended Cornell Medical College as a
Jonas Salk Scholar. Dr. Levitt interned and was a first-
year medical resident at Bellevue Hospital and then spent
2 years in the Public Health Service at the Encephalitis
Research Center in Tampa, Florida. He did his neurology
training at the Harvard teaching hospitals of the Longwood
Area Neurology Program.

With a Foreword by Charles F. Barlow, M.D.

Charles F. Barlow, M.D., is the Bronson Crothers Professor
of Neurology at Harvard Medical School, Neurologist-in-
Chief at Children's Hospital Medical Center, and serves as
Consultant in Neurology for the Brigham and Women's
Hospital, and Beth Israel Hospital. Since 1963, he has
been the Director of the Longwood Area Neurology Training
Program involving Children's Hospital Medical Center,

Brigham and Women's Hospital, and Beth Israel Hospital. His responsibilities include teaching of medical students, interns and residents, direction of the Mental Retardation and Human Development Research Program at Children's Hospital Medical Center, and care of children with neurologic disorders.

This manual is designed to guide house officers in recognizing and treating pediatric neurologic disease. It is not meant to be a complete survey, but an attempt to outline succinctly, important clinical information about common pediatric neurologic problems. This pediatric neurology manual is an outgrowth of a similar manual written for house officers of adult patients. The favorable response to the adult manual and the demand by our colleagues for a comparable one in pediatric neurology have been the impetus behind this book. As in the adult manual, we have tried to retain a problem-oriented approach wherever possible and hope the manual fills the need for a readable, "carry in the pocket," practical reference to the neurologic problems of pediatric patients.

Howard L. Weiner, M.D.
David K. Urion, M.D.
Lawrence P. Levitt, M.D.

Acknowledgments

This third edition was reviewed by residents in the Harvard-Longwood Area Neurology Training Program. We are grateful for their enthusiasm, advice, and thoughtful criticism, particularly with a view of those sections in the second edition that were in need of major overhaul. In particular, we wish to thank Drs. K. Daffner, H. Gelband, and H. Maguire for their special contributions in this light. We would also like to thank the following people for their help in the preparation of this third edition: Drs. C. Barlow, K. Kuban, and E. Kolodny.

Contents

Chapter 1

Localization

In pediatric neurology, the neurologic examination should answer two questions. (1) Is there a focal lesion in the nervous system? (2) Has the nervous system matured appropriately for the child's age?

During infancy and the first years of life, maturation and localization serve as dual fulcrums on which understanding lesions of the nervous system must hinge. As a child matures and the nervous system becomes more like an adult's, localization becomes the cornerstone of neurologic diagnosis.

//Where is the lesion? What is the lesion?//

Anatomic orientation is not merely an intellectual exercise; knowing where the lesion is is important in deciding on diagnostic procedures, will help guide in management, and will often lead to the diagnosis. For example:

Hypotonia: hypotonia is a nonspecific sign that can result from dysfunction at any point along the entire neuraxis: from cerebral cortex, through basal ganglia, cerebellum and spinal cord, to anterior horn cell, nerves, muscle, and even ligaments. For example, in Werdnig-Hoffmann disease (infantile spinal muscular atrophy), although motor milestones are markedly delayed, intellectual maturation is normal. The abnormality is of anterior horn cells in the spinal cord, not neurons in the cerebral cortex.

1

Spastic Diplegia: weakness of the lower extremities may be secondary to a lesion in the spinal cord (e.g., spinal cord tumor) or in the cerebral hemispheres (cerebral palsy, hydrocephalus).

Foot Drop: this may be seen with peripheral nerve (decreased deep tendon reflexes), spinal cord (increased deep tendon reflexes, sensory level), or hemispheres disease (increased deep tendon reflexes, cortical sensory loss, mental changes). Thus, one must localize the dysfunction before beginning investigation.

Ataxia: this is a common presenting sign in pediatrics. It is usually secondary to cerebellar disease (e.g., tumor, cerebellitis) but may be a false localizing sign since involvement of cerebellar connections (brainstem, thalamus, frontal lobes) can also cause ataxia. Ataxia is ipsilateral when the cerebellum is involved, whereas it is usually contralateral to involvement of its connections.

Crossed Signs: e.g., cranial nerve involvement on one side with corticospinal signs on the opposite side, localizes the lesion to the brainstem. In the spinal cord, crossed motor and sensory involvements are typical of unilateral cord involvement (Brown-Sequard syndrome).

Hysterical Symptoms and Signs: these are suspected when symptoms and signs do not fit anatomic rules. Beware of this diagnosis in children younger than 10 to 12 years old. Often they are more truly "conversion" phenomena, i.e., there is a kernel of truth in the complaints, but the child, not understanding them, or being fearful, elaborates them to the point of incapacity. Denial of failing vision is a common phenomenon in the younger child.

Suggested Readings

Haymaker W: Bing's Local Diagnosis in Neurological Disease. St. Louis, C.V. Mosby, 1969.
Maloney MJ: Diagnosing hysterical conversion reactions in children. J Pediatr 97:1016, 1980.

Chapter 2

Development

Developmental milestones are attained most rapidly during the 1st year of life; the infant's motor system, at first dependent primarily on brainstem and spinal cord, becomes influenced by the maturing cerebral hemispheres. Certain reflexes serve as important indices of nervous system maturation (Table 2.1).

REFLEXES AND SIGNS THAT DISAPPEAR

A. Moro Reflex: sudden abduction of the arms, extension of the legs, and flexion of the hips when the position of the head is changed abruptly in relationship to the body. The Moro reflex is present in all normal full term infants. It is an indicator of the symmetry and intactness of the nervous system, e.g., decreased Moro reflex on the side of a hemiparesis. It diminishes during the first months of life and usually disappears by 4 to 5 months.

B. Tonic Neck Reflex: with the infant supine, turning the head to one side results in extension of the arm and leg on that side with flexion of the contralateral arm, viz., a fencing posture. It is usually not present in the newborn but appears after 2 to 3 weeks. The reflex is most prominent during the 2nd month of life and infants may assume it spontaneously.

//An obligate or persistent tonic
neck reflex is abnormal.//

3

1. An <u>obligate</u> tonic neck reflex is always abnormal. After the infant's head is turned and he assumes the "fencing posture," a normal infant will "break" the posture after a few seconds. In an obligate response, the infant maintains the tonic neck posture as long as his head is turned to the side.

TABLE 2.1

REFLEXES AND SIGNS DURING THE 1ST YEAR

Reflex	Appears	Disappears
Moro	Birth	4-5 months
Stepping and placing	Birth	Persists as voluntary standing
Positive supporting	Newborn-3 months	Persists voluntarily
Tonic neck	2-3 weeks	4-6 months (never obligatory or sustained)
Crossed adductor	2-3 months	7-8 months
Neck righting	Begins 4-6 months	Persists voluntarily
Parachute	Begins 6-7 months	Persists
Grasp		
Palmar grasp (reflex)	Birth	3-4 months
Voluntary reach	4-5 months	
Palmar grasp (voluntary)	4-5 months (whole hand)	
	6-7 months (pincer)	

2. A consistently <u>asymmetrical</u> tonic neck response may be an early sign of hemiparesis on the side of the increased response.

3. The tonic neck reflex is rarely present after 5 to 6 months of age, and <u>persistence</u> after this time is abnormal. Sitting is usually impossible until this reflex disappears, and an obligate response precludes rolling over.

C. <u>Crossed Adductor Reflex</u>: contraction of both hip adductors when either knee jerk is elicited. The crossed adductor response usually disappears by 7 to 8 months of age, and persistence beyond that time is a sign of pyramidal tract dysfunction.

D. <u>Ankle Clonus</u>: (8 to 10 beats) may be present in the normal newborn but generally disappears by age 2 months.

E. The <u>Babinski</u> (extensor plantar) response is considered normal until 1 year of age, although this point is controversial. Some observers maintain the toe response is always flexor. We feel the Babinski response is abnormal during the first year only if it is repeatedly and easily elicitable, asymmetrical, or associated with other abnormal signs. In a normal baby, the plantar response may vary on successive trials and often fatigues rapidly.

NOTE: The <u>Chaddock maneuver</u> (stimulation of the dorsolateral aspect of the foot producing an upgoing toe) can be useful in infants and children in whom plantar stimulation results in plantar grasping or withdrawal. Similarly, contraction of the tensor facia lata may be useful in equivocal cases.

REFLEXES AND SIGNS THAT APPEAR

A. <u>Neck Righting Reflex</u>: with the infant supine, turning the head to one side causes the infant to turn his shoulders and trunk to the same side. It appears when the tonic neck reflex disappears, viz., at 4 months, when the baby begins to roll over. All normal infants have a neck righting reflex by age 8 to 10 months, after which it becomes part of voluntary activity.

B. Handgrasp: an infant is able to reach and grasp with his whole hand by 4 to 5 months of age. Thumb and finger (pincer) grasp begins at 6 to 7 months of age and is present in normal infants by 1 year. Transferring objects from one hand to the other begins at 7 to 8 months. A strong preference to use one hand is abnormal prior to 1 year of age when the first clear evidence of handedness appears. Ambidexterity in writing after age 3 is suspect.

C. Posture in Horizontal Suspension is a test of head control and motor function. At age 5 months, infants held horizontally (parallel to the floor) begin to arch their back and hold their head above the horizontal plane.

D. Posture in Vertical Suspension is flexor during the first half year of life. Persistent extension and adduction or "scissoring" of the lower extremities is always abnormal and a sign of spasticity. In the standing position, a normal positive supporting reaction consists of the child briefly bearing some weight. A "too good" positive supporting reaction is often the earliest sign of spasticity. In atonic diplegia, withdrawal of extremities and lack of a positive supporting reaction may be present. Withdrawal of extremities with hip flexion and knee extension is often described by families as "unwillingness" to bear weight.

E. Parachute Reflex: the infant is suspended horizontally and then plunged downward; the reflex consists of arm extension to "break the fall." It begins at 6 to 7 months and is well developed by 1 year. The parachute reflex is an excellent test of upper extremity pyramidal function and, if asymmetrical, may be a sign of hemiparesis.

OTHER DEVELOPMENTAL MILESTONES

Assessment of developmental milestones is best performmed with a standardized screening test. The Denver Developmental Screening Test (Fig. 25.12) outlines, in percentage form, gross motor, fine motor, language, and personal-social milestones over the first 6 years. When a child is able to use a pencil, Gesell, Binet, and Bender-Gestalt drawings (Fig. 2.1) are simple tests of fine motor and "conceptual" development. More definitive assessment is obtained by formal neuropsychological testing.

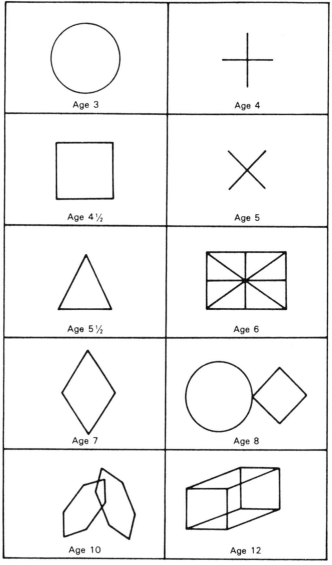

Figure 2.1   Ask child to copy figure appropriate for age.

A. <u>Walking</u>: most children walk well by age 14 to 15 months. If a child does not walk by 18 months, there is probably an abnormality (obesity is not a cause of late walking). When confronted with a child who is a late walker, check for:

1. <u>Clues to Neurologic Damage.</u>

a. Abnormal reflexes, e.g., Babinski's.
b. Head circumference below 3%.
c. History of perinatal distress.
d. Delayed speech.
e. Check creatinine phosphokinase to rule out dystrophy.
f. Check thyroid functions.

2. <u>Family History</u>: there are families in which late walking occurs as a normal variant.

B. <u>Language</u>: most children say single words by 14 months and combine words by 20 to 24 months. By age 2 years, a child should be able to combine two different words and point to a named body part. In a child with delayed language consider:

1. Clues to neurologic damage (above); <u>mental retardation</u> is the most common cause.

2. Hearing or visual deficit.

3. Autism.

4. Aphasia.

5. Oral motor problems (difficulty sucking, blowing, and excessive or prolonged drooling are all signs of an articulatory dyspraxia, especially where understanding outstrips expressive abilities).

> //Check hearing in a child with
> delayed language development.//

C. <u>Prematurity</u>: the premature infant may not attain developmental milestones as quickly as a full term infant. Nevertheless, a child born 4 weeks premature generally "catches up" by age 1 year.

D. <u>Systemic Illness</u>: normal developmental milestones may not apply to infants and children with significant

systemic illness, e.g., cardiac disease, cystic
fibrosis, and celiac disease.

NOTE: In newborns it is possible to estimate
          gestational age on the basis of physical and
          neurologic findings (J Pediatr 77:1, 1970).

Suggested Readings

        Illingworth RS: The Development of the Infant and
Young Child: Normal and Abnormal. London, Churchill
Livingstone, 1975.
        Paine RS, Brazelton BT, Donovan DE, et al: .
Evolution of postural reflexes in normal infants and in
the presence of chronic brain syndromes. Neurology
14:1036, 1964.
        Paine RS, Oppe, TE: Neurologic Examination of
Children. Clinics in Developmental Medicine, No. 20-21,
London, W. Heinemann, Spastics International Medical
Publications, No. 20-21, 1966.
        Ross ED, Velez-Borras J, Rosman NP: The
significance of the Babinski sign in the newborn - a
reappraisal. Pediatrics 57:13, 1976.

Chapter 3

The Hypotonic or Floppy Infant

Diagnosis requires establishing the level of nervous system dysfunction; hypotonia may result from a lesion of the cerebrum, spinal cord, peripheral nerve, myoneural junction, or muscle (Fig. 3.1).

IS THE LESION IN THE CEREBRUM?

1. Encephalopathy: damage to a normally formed brain. This is the most common cause of hypotonia (atonic forms of cerebral palsy). These infants usually have upgoing toes, especially with the Chaddock maneuver. The abnormality may be confined to the lower extremities in "atonic diplegia." Some children also have delayed social and language development. A careful history often reveals perinatal difficulties.

    //Atonic cerebral palsy is the most common neurologic cause of the floppy infant syndrome.//

2. Dysgenesis: an abnormally formed brain. These children may have obvious dysgenetic features (abnormal faces, fingers, and ear abnormalities) and may fit a recognizable syndrome, e.g., trisomy 21. (The Prader-Willi syndrome includes hypotonia, hypogonadism, hypomentia, obesity, and an abnormality of chromosome 15.)

3. Degenerative: regression of a normal nervous system. This category includes diseases such as Tay-Sachs disease, mucopolysaccharidoses, and amino acid disorders. A period of normal development, followed

12

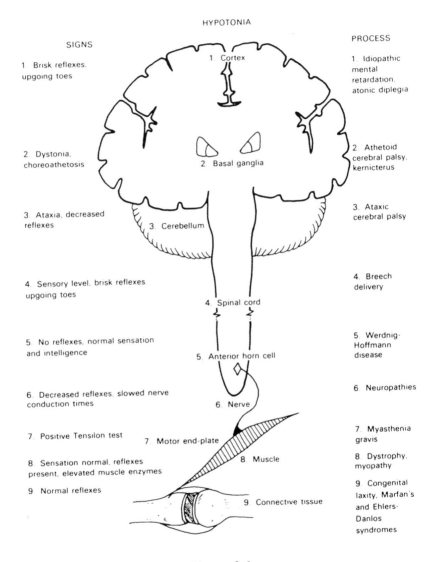

HYPOTONIA

SIGNS

1. Brisk reflexes,
upgoing toes

2. Dystonia,
choreoathetosis

3. Ataxia, decreased
reflexes

4. Sensory level, brisk reflexes
upgoing toes

5. No reflexes, normal sensation
and intelligence

6. Decreased reflexes, slowed nerve
conduction times

7. Positive Tensilon test

8. Sensation normal, reflexes
present, elevated muscle enzymes

9. Normal reflexes

PROCESS

1. Idiopathic
mental
retardation,
atonic diplegia

2. Athetoid
cerebral palsy,
kernicterus

3. Ataxic
cerebral palsy

4. Breech
delivery

5. Werdnig-
Hoffmann
disease

6. Neuropathies

7. Myasthenia
gravis

8. Dystrophy,
myopathy

9. Congenital
laxity, Marfan's
and Ehlers-
Danlos
syndromes

1. Cortex

2. Basal ganglia

3. Cerebellum

4. Spinal cord

5. Anterior horn cell

6. Nerve

7. Motor end-plate

8. Muscle

9. Connective tissue

Figure 3.1

by loss of milestones, is characteristic. Some
degenerative diseases, such as metachromatic
leukodystrophy, also affect peripheral nerves.

IS THE LESION IN THE SPINAL CORD?

1. <u>Spinal</u> <u>Cord</u> <u>Transection</u>: may present as hypotonia and
   usually occurs in association with a breech delivery.
   There may not be increased reflexes and upgoing toes,
   since acute cord injury can produce flaccid "spinal
   shock" lasting several weeks. Diagnosis is made by
   finding a sensory level to pin or sweat in the upper
   thoracic area, and a dilated bladder, and should be
   suspected when there is a positive birth history.
   Occasionally such transections can occur because of
   intrauterine fetal position, "star gazing fetus," and
   such infants should be delivered by cesarean section.
   Rarely, a transverse myelopathy will result from use
   of umbilical artery catheters.

2. <u>Spinal</u> <u>Cord</u> <u>Maldevelopment</u>: myelodysplasia,
   dysraphism, or incomplete closure of the neural tube
   (occult spina bifida, <u>not</u> myelomeningocele) is a
   developmental defect that affects the lumbar cord and
   produces lower extremity hypotonia, absence of some
   segmental deep tendon reflexes, and club feet; it is
   associated with vertebral abnormalities and
   occasionally skin anomalies (high placed pits, tuft of
   hair, nevus flammeus over the lumbosacral region).

IS THE LESION IN THE ANTERIOR HORN CELL?

1. <u>Werdnig-Hoffmann</u> <u>Disease</u> (infantile spinal muscular
   atrophy): affects anterior horn cells and produces
   hypotonia with absent reflexes. Although
   fasciculations are the hallmark of anterior horn cell
   disease, they are seldom seen in infants because of
   subcutaneous fat. They may be seen in the tongue,
   although the interpretation of a quivering tongue in a
   fussy infant is difficult. Finger tremors commonly
   seen in such infants may represent fasciculations.
   Diagnosis is made by muscle biopsy, which shows
   neurogenic atrophy. The disease may begin <u>in</u> <u>utero</u>
   (mother notices a decrease in fetal movements). The
   earlier the onset, the worse the prognosis. Some
   children die before age 1, while others survive into
   late teens. Benign variants with a later onset have
   been described (Kugelberg-Welander). A striking
   clinical feature is the intact cerebral function,

bright and inquisitive facies, and normal language development. Remember, a hypotonic infant with normal reflexes does not have Werdnig-Hoffmann disease.

2. Glycogen Storage Disease (type II - Pompe's): glycogen is deposited in anterior horn cells of brainstem and spinal cord; muscle dysfunction is also present. There is absent acid maltase; diagnosis is made by muscle biopsy and white blood cell (WBC) assay.

3. Poliomyelitis: now a rare cause of hypotonia. It presents with the abrupt onset of weakness, most often asymmetrically, in association with a febrile illness; spinal fluid is abnormal. Coxsackie virus is now an important cause of this syndrome.

IS THE LESION IN THE PERIPHERAL NERVE?

1. Polyneuropathy is a cause of hypotonia. Polyneuritis (Guillain-Barre) is uncommon in infants. Metachromatic and Krabbe's leukodystrophy affect peripheral nerves. Diagnosis of peripheral nerve dysfunction is based on slowed nerve conduction velocities and elevated cerebrospinal fluid protein.

IS THE LESION AT THE MYONEURAL JUNCTION?

1. Myasthenia Gravis may present as a floppy infant. This includes transient neonatal myasthenia in an infant of a myasthenic mother (occurs in 10% of myasthenics) or the much rarer congenital persistent myasthenia gravis. There is facial weakness, difficulty sucking and swallowing, and a weak cry. If the cause is unknown and myasthenia is suspected, pharmacologic testing with edrophonium is indicated.

2. Infant Botulism: this syndrome of acquired hypotonia, weakness, and respiratory distress has been described in infants during the first year of life. It appears to be secondary to absorption of toxin from clostridia organisms in the gut.

3. Toxic Neuromuscular Blockage secondary to "aminoglycoside" antibiotics, e.g., kanamycin, gentamycin, neomycin, may cause hypotonia, especially in children with renal failure. Hypermagnesemia is a cause of hypotonia in newborns secondary to treatment for pre-eclampsia.

IS THE LESION IN MUSCLE? (also see Chap. 16)

1. Congenital Structural Myopathies (nemaline, central core, and myotubular present as a floppy infant): diagnosis is made by muscle biopsy. There may be slow or no progression of symptoms in these myopathies.

2. Arthrogryposis Multiplex Congenita: this condition of joint contractures in the neonate is secondary to intrauterine hypotonia and lack of mobility. The underlying etiology must be sought by electromyogram (EMG), nerve conduction velocities, and muscle biopsy.

3. Myotonic Dystrophy: these children have poor sucking, facial diplegia (a "fish mouth"), and ptosis; they are usually mentally retarded. There is a positive family history, most often in the mother; percussion myotonia and a characteristic EMG come late.

4. Congenital Muscular Dystrophy is a rare cause of hypotonia. Diagnosis is made by biopsy. (The common dystrophies of childhood rarely present before age 2 to 3.)

SYSTEMIC CAUSES OF HYPOTONIA (Most significant acute and chronic systemic illnesses of childhood result in hypotonia, e.g., cyanotic congenital heart disease.)

1. Amino acid abnormalities.

2. Hypercalcemia.

3. Renal acidosis.

4. Rickets (may have an associated myopathy)/scurvy.

5. Hypothyroidism.

6. Celiac disease; cystic fibrosis.

7. Congenital laxity of ligaments - collagen dysfunction (Marfan and Ehlers-Danlos syndromes) and lysine hydrolase deficiency.

8. Failure to thrive/maternal deprivation.

BENIGN CONGENITAL HYPOTONIA (Amyotonia Congenita)

This diagnosis is made only after normal neuromuscular studies and long term follow-up. Some children in this category have residual clumsiness.

WORKUP

1. Urine analysis, electrolytes, thyroid studies, amino acid screen.

2. X-rays of spine and long bones. Computed axial tomographic (CAT) scan or magnetic resonance imaging (MRI) of brain where indicated (central causes).

3. Creatine phosphokinase.

4. Lumbar puncture.

5. EEG.

6. EMG, nerve conduction, muscle biopsy.

7. Urinary screen and WBC enzyme assays for degenerative disorders (e.g., mucopolysaccharidoses, metachromatic leukodystrophy, Tay-Sachs disease). These rare causes should be checked where indicated (see Chap. 10).

8. Edrophonium test when myasthenia is suspected.

9. Stool culture for clostridia.

The majority of children (75%) presenting with hypotonia between 6 months and 2 1/2 years have perinatal encephalopathy ("cerebral palsy") or idiopathic mental and motor retardation; the remainder have one of the other causes discussed above.

Genetic counseling is important for certain causes of hypotonia and is a major reason for pursuing a complete workup of the hypotonic or floppy infant.

Suggested Readings

Argov Z, Mastaglia FL: Disorders of neuromuscular transmission caused by drugs. N Engl J Med 301:409-413, 1979.

Dubowitz V: Muscle Disorders in Childhood, Vol 15 of Major Problems in Clinical Pediatrics. Philadelphia, W.B. Saunders, 1978.

Dubowitz V: The Floppy Infant, 2nd ed. Clinics in Developmental Medicine, No. 76. London, W. Heinemann, Spastics International Medical Publications, 1980.

Dubowitz V, Brooke MH: Muscle biopsy: a modern approach. In Major Problems in Neurology, vol 2. Philadelphia, W.B. Saunders, 1973.

Fenishel GM: Clinical syndromes of myasthenia in infancy and childhood. Arch Neurol 35:97, 1978.

Johnson RO: Diagnosis and management of infant botulism. Am J Dis Child 133:586, 1979.

Myers GJ: Understanding the floppy baby. Adv Neurol 17:295, 1977.

Paine RS: The future of the floppy infant: a follow-up study of 133 patients. Dev Med Child Neurol 5:115, 1963.

Snead OC, et al: Juvenile myasthenia gravis. Neurology 30:732, 1980.

Chapter 4

Cerebral Palsy

"Cerebral palsy" (perinatal encephalopathy) is a fixed, nonprogressive neurologic deficit acquired before, during, or in the months after birth. Cerebral palsy is a description, not a diagnosis. Although it is a useful term, the physician should if possible indicate the etiology, e.g., cerebral palsy secondary to neonatal meningitis. Despite the nonprogressive nature of damage, the clinical expression of cerebral palsy may change as the child matures. The approach to the child with possible cerebral palsy is first the elimination of progressive processes as diagnostic possibilities and then the application of a transdisciplinary approach to the care of the child.

HISTORY AND PHYSICAL EXAMINATION

1. Establish the history surrounding the mother's pregnancy and delivery. Was the baby premature or "small for dates"? Did the mother see the child immediately after birth? Was there a low Apgar score? Did the child leave the hospital on time? Was there blood group incompatibility producing jaundice? Was the baby tube fed? Was oxygen or a respirator needed?

2. Were there seizures, meningitis, or major illnesses during the first months of the child's life?

3. Is there evidence of spasticity (increased tone, hyperactive reflexes, upgoing toes)? Was there hypotonia during the 1st year of life?

4. Are there persistent infantile reflexes, e.g., tonic neck reflexes?

5. Did the parents notice the child favoring one hand before age 12 months?

6. Is one limb or hand smaller than the other? Check thumbnail and toenail sizes for discrepancies in square area.

7. Is there evidence of a movement disorder such as (a) athetosis: turning or twisting of an extremity; (b) chorea: quick jerks of an extremity, hand, or finger; or (c) dystonia: heightened tone and abnormal posture in an extremity, the trunk maintained in a unnatural position, e.g., head turned to the side, leg turned in? These may be brought out by having the child run or carry out other motor activity.

8. Is there evidence of other congenital abnormalities? Is there strabismus?

9. Is there macro- or microcephaly?

10. Establish developmental milestones and concordance of developmental and chronologic age.

TYPES OF CEREBRAL PALSY

A. Spastic Diplegia: increased tone and spasticity in the legs. Damage is acquired in utero or at birth, often secondary to anoxia, acidosis, and hypotension; it is more common in premature than full term infants. The diplegia may be seen during the 1st year of life in a child with marked cerebral damage or it may be a subtle finding in an otherwise normal older child. Severely affected children have quadriplegia, are mentally retarded, have difficulty speaking and swallowing, and have a tendency to drool; some never walk.

Features of Diplegia Include:

1. Adduction, extension, and internal rotation of the legs. This causes a characteristic "scissoring" of the legs when the child is suspended.

2. Tightened heel cords.

3. Increased tone and reflexes in the lower extremities, often with ankle clonus and upgoing toes.

4. There may be clumsiness and abnormal posturing in the upper extremities. There are no sphincter disturbances.

The infant comes to the pediatrician because of delayed motor milestones, the older child because of gait abnormalities. Differential diagnosis of spasticity primarily in the legs includes: (1) a local spinal cord process, e.g., tumor; (2) hydrocephalus, causing periventricular stretching of leg fibers; and (3) parasagittal intracranial mass. Treatment includes physical therapy and, in severe diplegia, heel cord lengthening and adductor myotomies. Many children with spastic diplegia have normal intelligence. Spastic diplegia may result from parasagittal "border zone" lesions (i.e., the maximum brunt of the damage occurs in the area between major cerebral vessels) or from periventricular leukomalacia (i.e., focal areas of white matter necrosis constitute a pattern of damage peculiar to the neonate and its normally unmyelinated hemispheres). Both are associated with perinatal anoxia, hypotension, acidosis, and sepsis.

B. Spastic Hemiplegia refers to spasticity in arm and leg. It is caused by a unilateral insult, e.g., head trauma, vascular event, or congenital abnormality, occurring in utero, at birth, or during the first months of life. Spastic hemiplegia is the most common form of cerebral palsy acquired after birth. When congenital, the hemiparesis is often not recognized by parents until age 4 to 12 months when the child favors one side or is slow in attaining developmental milestones. Initially, the affected side is flaccid and hyporeflexic; it later becomes hypertonic and spastic. Unless there is severe intellectual impairment, most children learn to walk. One-half walk by age 18 months, two-thirds by 2 years, and 90% by 36 months. Many children have an associated strabismus. Underdevelopment of the affected side is common, check thumbnail and toenail sizes. Normal intelligence is seen in one-third of the children; mental retardation is more common in those with a seizure disorder. Physical therapy is used to help prevent contractures, and orthopaedic surgery may be needed.

C. <u>Extrapyramidal</u> <u>Cerebral</u> <u>Palsy</u>: these children present
with slow motor development. They are seen at 10 to
18 months of age because they are unable to sit;
righting and tonic neck reflexes are prominent and
there may be drooling. In infancy, there is hypotonia
and easily obtained reflexes. As the infant grows
older, choreoathetosis and dystonia develop. The
majority learn to walk, although it may take 2 to 3
years after they learn to sit. The presence of an
obligatory tonic neck response and prominent righting
reflexes lessens the chance of sitting and walking.
Children with extrapyramidal cerebral palsy are
frequently not retarded and do not have seizures. In
the past, kernicterus has been a significant cause of
extrapyramidal cerebral palsy. In these cases hearing
should be tested. Pathologically, <u>status</u> <u>marmoratus</u>
(marble-like scarring in the basal ganglia) has been
found in extrapyramidal cerebral palsy.

Some children with spastic cerebral palsy at birth may
develop extrapyramidal features late in the 1st or
early in the 2nd decade. "Cerebellar" cerebral palsy
is very rare. It is characterized by hypotonia,
decreased reflexes, and ataxia. The etiology is most
often a cerebellar dysgenesis/dysplasia.

TREATMENT

The approach to the child with cerebral palsy is
transdisciplinary. The pediatrician must rule out
entities such as tumor or degenerative disease. Physical
therapy is needed to prevent contractures and maximize
motor abilities in children with spasticity. Braces are
often helpful. In some instances heel cord lengthening
and adductor myotomies are of benefit. Psychological
testing is necessary to evaluate intellectual abilities
and aid in proper school placement. Remember, the
spectrum of cerebral palsy is wide, ranging from severely
retarded children who cannot walk to those with normal
intelligence and mild motor deficits.

Suggested Readings

Christensen E, Melchior J: Cerebral Palsy, A Clinical
and Neuropathological Study. <u>Clinics</u> <u>in</u> <u>Developmental</u>
<u>Medicine</u>, No. 25. London, W. Heinemann, 1967.
Crothers B, Paine RS: <u>The</u> <u>Natural</u> <u>History</u> <u>of</u> <u>Cerebral</u>
<u>Palsy</u>. Cambridge, Harvard University Press, 1959.

Friede RL: Developmental Neuropathology. New York, Springer-Verlag, 1975.

Kuban K, Gilles FH: Human telencephalic angiogenesis. Ann Neurol 17:6, 1985.

Leviton A, Gilles FH: Acquired perinatal leukoencephalopathy. Ann Neurol 61:1, 1984.

Nelson KB, Ellenberg JH: Neonatal signs as predictors of cerebral palsy. Pediatrics 64:225, 1979.

Volpe J: Neurology of the Newborn, vol. 12 of Major Problems in Clinical Pediatrics. Philadelphia, W.B. Saunders, 1981.

Chapter 5

Macrocephaly

Of all the measurements taken by a pediatrician, head circumference may be of greatest importance. However, it is frequently omitted, especially after the first few months of life. A normal increase in skull size reflects a growing brain; when the skull becomes too large (see head circumference charts, Figs. 25.10 and 25.11), there usually is underlying intracranial pathology. Most children with abnormally large heads have either hydrocephalus or subdural collections of fluids. Rarely, megalencephaly (excessive brain mass) may be the cause of an enlarged head. Some of these children have a progressive degeneration associated with accumulation of abnormal substrates, e.g., Tay-Sachs disease, Alexander's disease, or Canavan's disease. Megalencephaly may also be associated with one of the phakomatoses, especially neurofibromatosis. Others are idiopathic or dysgenetic; some may be familial. Remember to measure head circumferences of other family members.

CLINICAL EVALUATION

1. Serial measurement will identify a head that is growing rapidly. Yet, not all rapidly growing heads require immediate study. If the child is asymptomatic, he can be followed until several percentile lines are crossed and occasionally beyond the 97th percentile. Rapid head growth may occur normally in premature infants and is seen in older infants after a period of starvation.

2. Skull shape may provide a clue to the underlying
   condition: (a) Parietal bulging in porencephaly and
   subdural fluid collections. (b) Bilateral frontal
   prominence in obstructive hydrocephalus. There may or
   may not be a "setting sun" sign (downward deviation of
   the eyes). (c) A small posterior fossa in aqueductal
   stenosis. (d) A prominent occiput in posterior fossa
   cysts.

3. Palpably split sutures and a bulging fontanelle may
   occur in infants with raised intracranial pressure.
   In addition, the anterior fontanelle can be used to
   estimate intracranial pressure in infants by
   determining the height above the heart at which it
   flattens. In a quiet, sitting infant the fontanelle
   is flat and pulsating. In children with increased
   intracranial pressure and a closed fontanelle, a
   "cracked pot" sound may be heard on percussion of the
   skull.

4. Careful transillumination: in total darkness, a
   flashlight with a rubber adapter is tightly applied to
   all areas of the skull. An area of illumination in
   excess of 2.5 cm is abnormal. Diffuse
   transillumination is seen with hydranencephaly
   (congenital absence of cortical tissue), severe
   hydrocephalus with marked thinning of the cerebral
   mantle, bilateral subdural effusions, and occasionally
   in diffuse cerebral atrophy with enlarged subarachnoid
   spaces. Asymmetrical supratentorial transillumination
   may be associated with subdural effusion,
   porencephaly, or unilateral ventricular dilation.
   Posterior fossa transillumination, especially if
   midline and triangular, suggests a Dandy-Walker
   malformation of the cerebellum; asymmetrical posterior
   fossa transillumination is seen with subarachnoid
   cysts. Subdural collections of blood do not
   transilluminate.

A normal skull transilluminates more in the frontal
region. Skulls of premature infants transilluminate more
than those of full term infants. Beware of false
transillumination from extravasated intravenous fluids in
the scalp.

LABORATORY STUDIES

In addition to CAT scan, the evaluation of
macrocephaly should include skull x-rays. A bulging

anterior fontanelle may be seen on plain x-rays. In the older child, thinning of the floor of the sella may precede separation of sutures, which is rarely seen in children over 13 years of age. Other changes include a small posterior fossa in aqueductal stenosis and asymmetrical thinning of bones overlying cysts. The CAT scan is particularly useful in identifying cysts and hydrocephalus. Subdural taps and, in some instances, arteriography may be used to diagnose subdural collections of fluid. Contrast and other studies are occasionally required to diagnose the source of hydrocephalus accurately.

Note: Studies of head growth in premature infants indicate that they regularly cross percentiles during the first 3 months of life. The most rapid rates of head growth are observed in the smallest premature infants. The head of a healthy premature infant grows at 1.1 cm per week, i.e., twice the normal rate; after 2 months the rate falls to normal. It is important to use appropriate charts for pre- and post-term (40 weeks) growth.

MICROCEPHALY

Microcephaly is associated with genetic defects, chromosomal abnormalities, and neonatal or perinatal insults (infection, trauma, anoxia, radiation, and metabolic derangements such as the infantile forms of Krabbe's disease and metachromatic leukodystrophy). Whatever the cause, there is a high correlation between microcephaly (head size more than 2 standard deviations below normal) and mental retardation. Except for cases where there is craniosynostosis, small head size indicates a small brain.

HYDROCEPHALUS

Hydrocephalus is not a disease, but a symptom complex that results from any process that causes excessive accumulation of cerebrospinal fluid (CSF) in the ventricular system. The diagnosis of hydrocephalus requires demonstration of ventricular enlargement; enlargement results from impaired circulation and/or absorption of CSF and only in the rarest of cases, overproduction (choroid plexus papilloma). The clinical picture depends on the underlying cause and the age of the child. There may be irritability and failure to achieve milestones in the infant or signs of increased intracranial pressure (headache, vomiting, and

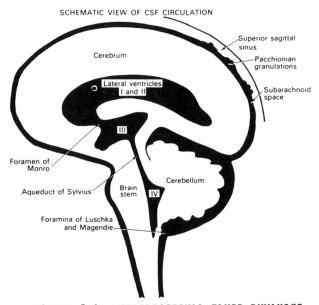

26

papilledema) in an older child. Spastic weakness of the lower extremities is often present, secondary to impingement on leg fibers by enlarged lateral ventricles. Many children are asymptomatic until the hydrocephalus becomes marked. In the neonate, head growth may lag behind developing hydrocephalus.

Hydrocephalus may be communicating or noncommunicating.

SCHEMATIC VIEW OF CSF CIRCULATION

Figure 5.1.   CEREBROSPINAL FLUID DYNAMICS

CSF is produced in the choroid plexus which is found in the lateral, third, and fourth ventricles. CSF flows from lateral ventricles through the foramen of Monro into the third ventricle, then through the aqueduct of Sylvius to the fourth ventricle. It exits from the fourth ventricle through the foramina of Luschka (lateral) and Magendie (medial) into the cisterns surrounding the cerebellum. From there it communicates with the entire subarachnoid space and drains mainly via pacchionian granulations into the superior sagittal sinus. Noncommunicating hydrocephalus implies a block somewhere between lateral ventricle and the foramina in the fourth ventricle.

Communicating hydrocephalus implies impaired absorption of CSF from the subarachnoid space.

A. Communicating is the most common type. CSF circulation from choroid plexus, via the ventricular system and to the posterior fossa foramina, is normal (Fig. 5.1). The block to absorption occurs somewhere in the subarachnoid space. Communicating hydrocephalus may be congential or acquired, e.g., acquired after meningitis or secondary to blood in the subarachnoid space (subarachnoid hemorrhage).

B. Noncommunicating implies a block at some level within the ventricular system, e.g., foramen of Monro, aqueduct of Sylvius, or the fourth ventricular foramina. Causes include congenital malformations, tumor, and, rarely, inflammatory conditions.

1. Congenital

a. Spina Bifida: Myelomeningocele:
Myelomeningocele is frequently associated with hydrocephalus, usually due to Chiari malformation (a maldevelopment with displacement of brainstem and cerebellar tonsils through the foramen magnum into the spinal canal) and/or aqueductal stenosis. Hydrocephalus may not be evident at birth in such infants. Significant hydrocephalus at birth, high thoracic cord lesions, and flaccid paraplegia are poor prognostic signs. The advisability of surgical intervention in these severely involved children is controversial. Future children of families with myelomeningocele are at increased risk, and prenatal diagnosis is possible by finding increased levels of alpha-fetoprotein in the amniotic fluid and in mother's blood.

b. Aqueductal Stenosis or Obstruction: aqueductal stenosis occurs secondary to malformations of the aqueduct or postinflammatory gliosis. The hydrocephalus may appear from the neonatal period to later childhood. The latter cases are usually "compensated," but decompensation may occur after a trivial insult, such as minor head trauma or infection.

c. Posterior Fossa Subarachnoid Cysts obstruct CSF flow in the region of the foramina of Luschka and Magendie. The Dandy-Walker syndrome consists of midline cerebellar agenesis and an associated cyst of the fourth ventricle; the occipital bone is prominent and triangular occipital transillumination is present.

d. Aneurysmal Dilation of the Vein of Galen causes obstruction by external pressure on the aqueduct and may be associated with high output cardiac failure in the infant.

2. Tumor: hydrocephalus occurs with posterior fossa tumors, particularly medulloblastoma and astrocytoma of the cerebellum. Brainstem gliomas cause hydrocephalus late in their course. Supratentorial tumors may cause obstruction at any level. Blood in the CSF of a child with hydrocephalus suggests a tumor.

DIAGNOSIS

After plain skull x-rays, CAT scan is the first step in evaluating and diagnosing children with hydrocephalus. In some instances, clear delineation of CSF pathways may require CAT scan, MRI, or contrast ventriculography. Cerebral angiography may be useful in evaluating children with hydrocephlus secondary to posterior fossa processes because it does not upset the equilibrium of the CSF. Lumbar puncture is hazardous in hydrocephalus and may cause decompensation.

In the very young infant and neonate, two-dimensional ultrasound has proven to be a very sensitive diagnostic tool for hydrocephalus.

TREATMENT

Although treatment must be individualized, shunting is an integral part of therapy in most situations. Shunts can be placed that connect the cerebral ventricles to the heart, pleural cavity, or peritoneum. Unfortunately, shunts frequently malfunction and/or become infected. In addition, they need to be lengthened with somatic growth. In the premature neonate, repeated lumbar puncture may allow postponement of shunting procedures until a more optimal time.

SUBDURAL COLLECTIONS OF FLUID

Subdural effusions (clear or xanthochromic fluid with an elevated protein) and hematoma are common in the first

2 years of life. Hematomas and effusions may be acute, subacute, or chronic. Effusions usually evolve from hematomas. Although hematomas are commonly associated with trauma, hematomas and/or effusions also occur in meningitis, dehydration (especially hypernatremic), leukemia, hemophilia, vitamin C and K deficiencies, after pneumoencephalography, and after shunting for hydrocephalus. Hematomas follow rupture of bridging veins in the potential subdural space, and blood causes the formation of an outer vascular and an inner avascular membrane. The clot usually liquifies and with the formation of the outer membrane, there is a continual leak of albumin and water into the space from new permeable blood vessels.

Subdural hematoma or effusion in infancy represents a special clinical entity, different from the acute subdural hematoma seen after head trauma in older children and adults. This latter syndrome consists of acute deterioration following the injury, with progressive neurologic dysfunction and focal signs. In infants, the progression of symptoms is less acute and there may be signs and symptoms as nonspecific as irritability and anemia. Diagnosis and treatment are straightforward, as subdural taps can be performed on the ward. Seizures are a common symptom; seizures and an enlarged head in an infant represent a subdural hematoma until proven otherwise.

//Macrocephaly and seizures suggest a subdural hematoma.//

Symptoms of subdural hematoma:

- Convulsions

- Vomiting

- Lethargy - stupor, coma

Signs associated with subdural hematoma:

- Enlarging head - bulging fontanelle

- Retinal hemorrhages

- Signs of external trauma

- Focal or bilateral abnormal neurologic signs, e.g., bilateral hyperreflexia, hemiparesis

. Positive transillumination only if subacute (blood does not transilluminate)

Although head trauma is an important factor in infantile subdural hematoma, a history of head trauma is often lacking and few infants have a skull fracture. The "battered child" syndrome should be kept in mind and a search should be made for other fractures (skeletal survey). Retinal hemorrhages in the first 6 months of life without evidence of external trauma strongly suggest the "whiplash-shaken infant" syndrome (Pediatrics 54:396, 1974). Head enlargement is usually parietal rather than frontal as in hydrocephalus.

Subdural effusions are characterized by the same symptoms and signs as hematomas, although the evolution is slower; effusion may be found in the workup of hydrocephalus. The following additional features may characterize effusions:

. Failure to thrive

. Developmental retardation

. Anemia

Up to 50% of infants with meningitis have effusions. Most are asymptomatic and do not require drainage.

Subdural hematoma in the neonate should be considered when an infant is doing poorly without obvious cause, particularly if there are seizures. The presentation is subacute with onset of symptoms in the 2nd week of life, beginning with vomiting and seizures and followed by skull enlargement. Acute subdurals-those producing symptoms within 1 to 3 days of birth-are rare and usually occur after markedly traumatic deliveries.

Posterior fossa subdurals (retrocerebellar) are a rare occurrence in the 1st week of life. The clinical picture includes enlarging head, nystagmus, breathing difficulties, and decerebration. Subdural taps of the frontal parietal area are negative, but the CSF is usually bloody. Posterior fossa subdurals are usually seen on CAT scan, but angiography may be necessary for diagnosis. Treatment is urgent and consists of surgical drainage. Posterior fossa subdural hematoma may occur in older children.

DIAGNOSIS AND TREATMENT

Whenever a symptomatic subdural hematoma is suspected (increasing lethargy, focal neurologic signs, persistent fever suggesting empyema), a prompt <u>subdural</u> <u>tap</u> should be carried out; this is both a diagnostic and a therapeutic maneuver. Tapping the subdural space through the anterior fontanelle or coronal suture can be done on the ward by someone with experience:

1. The child is immobilized, the head is shaved, and the skin is cleaned.

2. A short beveled 20-gauge needle with stylet is introduced at the lateral angle of the fontanelle (if greater than 3 cm from midline) or through the coronal suture (in line with the pupil).

3. When the dura is penetrated, a recognizable "pop" is felt. The needle should not be rotated and suction should not be applied.

4. A few drops of clear fluid may be obtained normally from the subarachnoid space, and this may be as much as 2 ml.

5. Check the protein level in fluid from the subdural tap against CSF obtained at lumbar puncture if the nature of the subdural fluid is uncertain.

Each day 15 ml/side may be removed and many collections of fluid will resolve within 10 to 14 days. The fluid is monitored with serial hematocrits; removal of large volumes may cause anemia and hypoproteinemia.
CAT scan usually demonstrates subdural collections of fluid, especially acute ones. It may miss chronic or small collections, especially those in the parasagittal area.
Cerebral arteriography almost always demonstrates subdural collections of fluid. Radioisotope brain scans may show increased uptake over the hemispheres and the EEG may show slowing or low voltage on the side of the subdural hematoma.
Traditionally, persistent collections of fluid have been treated by membrane stripping at craniotomy. Evidence indicates that membranes rarely constrict brain

growth, so less active measures, e.g., constant drainage and subdural peritoneal shunts, have also been employed.

The degree of cortical atrophy present at the time of treatment and the etiology of the collection correlate with subsequent intellectual deficits and epilepsy.

Suggested Readings

Bell WE, McCormick WF: Increased Intracranial Pressure in Children, 2nd ed, vol 8 of Major Problems in Clinical Pediatrics. Philadelphia, W.B. Saunders 1978.

Day RE, Schultz WH: Normal children with large heads – benign familial megalencephaly. Arch Dis Child 54:512, 1979.

Demyer W: Megalencephaly in children. Neurology 22:634, 1972.

Ferguson-Smith MA, Rawlinson HA, May HM, et al: Avoidance of anencephalic and spina bifida births by maternal serum-alphafetoprotein screening. Lancet 1:1330, 1978.

Fishman MA: Recent clinical advances in the treatment of dysraphic states. Pediatr Clin North Am 23:517, 1976.

Fishman RA: Cerebrospinal Fluid in Diseases of the Nervous System, Philadelphia, W.B. Saunders, 1980.

Lorber J: Results of treatment of myelomeningocele. Dev Med Child Neurol 13:279, 1971.

Matson DD: Neurosurgery of Infancy and Childhood. Springfield, IL, Charles C Thomas, 1969.

Shurtletf DB, Hayden PW, Loeser JD, Kronmal RA: Myelodysplasia: decision for death or disability. N Engl J Med 291:1005, 1974.

Chapter 6

Seizures

TYPES OF SEIZURES

Seizures are categorized by EEG into two major groups, depending on the source of the discharge: focal and primary generalized. In focal seizures (Fig. 6.1) the initial discharge comes from a focal unilateral area of the brain, e.g., temporal lobe, frontal lobe, motor strip. Thus, a child whose seizure begins with his right hand shaking has a focal seizure disorder attributable to a discharge originating in the frontal lobe. Focal seizure disorders are usually secondary to focal pathology, e.g., trauma, tumor, vascular abnormality, old scar, and mesial temporal lobe sclerosis.

In primary generalized seizures (Fig. 6.1) the discharge arises from deep midline structures in the brainstem or thalamus (which have direct and widespread connections to the cortex). This area is sometimes referred to as the "centrencephalon." There usually is no aura and there are no focal features during the seizure. An example of a primary generalized or "centrencephalic" seizure disorder is an absence attack (petit mal). A grand mal seizure is a major motor seizure involving all extremities and having both tonic and clonic features. It may be a generalized seizure from the onset (idiopathic epilepsy), or it can begin focally and then generalize to become grand mal (Fig. 6.1). This may happen so quickly that it is impossible to see the focality clinically, and the patient can recall no aura. Nonetheless, the EEG usually shows the focality and the seizure is classified as focal with secondary generalization.

Major motor seizures may occur in previously normal children secondary to metabolic factors, e.g., hypoglycemia. These are nonfocal seizures, not classified as "generalized" and not felt to represent a true epileptic disorder.

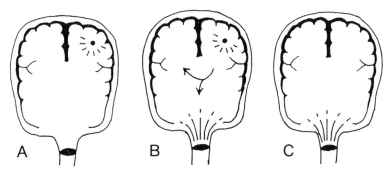

FIGURE 6.1 Classification of seizure disorders. A. Focal seizure beginning from a focal, unilateral part of the brain (e.g., right-sided tonic movements, eyes deviated to one side, or an automatism of temporal lobe epilepsy). B. Focal seizure with secondary generalization. Focal seizures may activate central centrencephalic structures or spread to the other side, resulting in a bilateral generalized convulsion. The seizure disorder is still classified as a focal one even though the focal element may have been transitory before the generalization. Most seizure disorders are focal, and almost all children whose seizures begin before age 3 or after age 18 have focal seizure disorder. (EEG usually shows the focality.) C. Primary generalized seizure. No focal component is present either clinically or on EEG. These seizures represent true "idiopathic epilepsy" (e.g., petit mal).

ESTABLISH THE "FOCALITY" OR "GENERALITY" OF THE DISORDER

History

1. Exactly how did the seizure start? Find a witness.
   Did the head and eyes turn? Were there other focal
   features? Sometimes the child can recall events at
   the beginning of the seizure if it was focal.

2. At what age did the seizure begin? True
   centrencephalic seizures rarely begin before age 3 or
   after age 18.

3. Is there a family history of seizures? This may be
   present in both types but is more characteristic of
   centrencephalic seizure disorders.

4. Was there focal trauma at birth or during an accident
   (head trauma)? Is there any history of previous
   neurologic insult (e.g., meningitis)?

5. Does the child have abdominal pains, nausea,
   dizziness, behavioral disturbances, or automatisms
   (frequent features of temporal lobe epilepsy)?

6. Have there been brief staring spells not followed by
   postictal confusion or fatigue (petit mal epilepsy,
   i.e., absence attacks)?

A Search for Focal or Generalized Features

1. When examining a child after a seizure, look for
   postictal paralysis (Todd's paralysis), i.e., check
   for asymmetry of reflexes, hemiparesis, upgoing toes,
   and hemiparetic posturing of a foot (everted).

2. Are the eyes tonically deviated during the seizure?
   For example, a left hemisphere seizure drives the eyes
   to the right. Following a seizure, however, they may
   be deviated toward the discharging hemisphere.

3. Look for asymmetry of fingernail, toe, and limb size
   (the smaller size of one limb may be a clue to early
   damage of the contralateral hemisphere).

4. Arteriovenous malformations may present as focal
   seizures: listen for a cranial bruit.

5. Petit mal (a centrencephalic seizure disorder) can be precipitated by hyperventilation. Have the child hyperventilate for 1 minute or longer.

6. Check skin for evidence of a phakomatosis (see Chap. 24). They are associated with focal lesions in the central nervous system.

SPECIFIC SEIZURE TYPES IN CHILDHOOD

Grand Mal Epilepsy/Generalized Epilepsy

A grand mal seizure is a major motor seizure involving all extremities and having both tonic and clonic features. Some children suffer grand mal attacks with no focal element, either during the attack or on EEG and there is no history of previous neurologic insult. These children suffer from idiopathic grand mal epilepsy, a genetically determined centrencephalic seizure disorder. Often a grand mal seizure represents a focal seizure that has generalized. In these instances there are usually focal discharges on EEG and the etiology of the seizure is a focal area of pathology. Initial treatment in both types of grand mal seizures is phenobarbital and/or phenytoin.

Temporal Lobe Epilepsy; Pyschomotor Seizures (focal or partial seizures with complex symptomatology)

This focal seizure disorder is secondary to a lesion in the temporal lobe. Causes include birth trauma, prolonged "febrile" convulsions, tumor, and hamartomas. There may be an aura prior to the seizure, often visceral, e.g., abdominal pains, "butterflies" in the stomach, and "funny feelings." The seizure itself may take the form of automatic movements such as swallowing or lip smacking, a repetitive motion with the hands (picking at one's clothes), behavior abnormalities (walking to another part of the room), or lack of responsiveness. There usually is amnesia for the episodes, postictal confusion, and drowsiness; temporal lobe seizures may generalize into grand mal attacks. Treatment includes phenytoin, phenobarbital, carbamazepine (Tegretol), and primidone (Mysoline). Remember, optic radiations course through the temporal lobe and supply the upper outer quadrant of vision; a superior quadrantanopsia may be the first sign of an expanding process in the temporal lobe. A sleep EEG may be needed to demonstrate discharges of temporal lobe epilepsy, and nasopharyngeal or anterior temporal lead recordings are useful when routine awake/sleep EEGs are negative.

Petit Mal Epilepsy: Absence Attacks

Petit mal epilepsy does not mean a child is having "small seizures"; it refers to a specific clinical phenomenon with unique and characteristic EEG findings (3 per second spike and wave discharges). It is an idiopathic, centrencephalic seizure disorder and is usually not associated with underlying structural pathology. Clinically, the absence attacks (often hundreds per day) consist of staring spells, mild ptosis, or eye fluttering that lasts seconds; usually there are no gross body movements, but automatisms can occur causing confusion with temporal lobe epilepsy. If seen at close range, blinking and nystagmus of the eyes are present and their rate may correlate with the 3 per second EEG. There is no postictal drowsiness. A child with continual discharges (petit mal status) may appear drugged but is usually able to walk and even speak ("petit mal stupor"). Petit mal epilepsy occurs almost exclusively between the ages of 4 and puberty. Approximately 75% of affected children will "outgrow" their petit mal seizures by puberty, and almost all do so by the beginning of the 3rd decade. Some children have, in addition, grand mal seizures. These children are less likely to outgrow their epilepsy, and there may be some atypical features on their EEGs. Petit mal attacks may be precipitated by hyperventilation, a maneuver carried out during EEG recording and when examining a child suspected of having petit mal. Ethosuximide (Zarontin) is the drug of choice. Valproic acid (Depakene) is also highly effective in pure petit mal, but ranks after ethosuximide because of potential toxic side effects, need for ancillary laboratory tests, and drug expense. Acetazolamide (Diamox) is a particularly useful adjunct drug in petit mal. A child should be given concomitant treatment with phenobarbital or phenytoin if there are major motor seizures or atypical features on EEG. Temporal lobe epilepsy is often misdiagnosed as petit mal (Table 6.1).

Table 6.1

DIFFERENTIAL FEATURES OF TEMPORAL LOBE AND PETIT MAL
SEIZURES

Feature	Temporal lobe	Petit mal
EEG	Focal discharge	3 per second spikes
Automatism	Present	Occasionally
Post-ictal drowsiness	Present	None
Frequency	Several per day	Hundreds occur daily
Age of onset	Occurs at any age	Predominantly ages 4-5 to puberty
Duration	Attack usually longer than 1 minute	Attack usually less than 30 seconds
Hyperventilation induced	Rarely	Frequently

Infantile Spasms and Hypsarrhythmia

Infantile spasms (salaam attacks) usually begin at
age 3 to 9 months. They may be mistaken for colic, and it
may be necessary to see an episode to make the diagnosis.
Most spasms are flexor in nature (like a Moro response);

//Infantile spasms may mimic colic.//

others may be extensor or involve only flexion of the
neck. Often there is an associated cry. Observation of an
infantile spasm is aided by having the baby relaxed, just
about to nap, or about to wake up. These spells are
associated with a very abnormal EEG pattern: disorganized
background, irregular high voltage slowing, multifocal
sharp waves, polyspikes, and burst suppression
(hypsarrhythmia).
The causes of this syndrome are diverse and the
spasms represent an age-specific seizure pattern generated
by an immature nervous system in response to diffuse

central nervous system (CNS) disease. Infantile spasms
may be symptomatic, occurring in infants with a history of
previous CNS difficulties or with overt CNS signs, or
cryptogenic, occurring in infants with normal examination
and no previous neurologic symptoms. The prognosis is
ominous: over 90% of such infants are ultimately retarded
and usually have a mixed, myoclonic-akinetic and
generalized seizure disorder after the age of 2 years.

A normal infant (cryptogenic group) with a normal
sized head who begins having spasms has the best
prognosis. If head growth slows or ceases with the onset
of spasms, the prognosis is poor.

Tuberous sclerosis may present as infantile
spasms; the diagnosis is made by finding ash leaf
depigmented spots, which may only be visible with
ultraviolet light (Wood's lamp).

Although there is no satisfactory treatment,
adrenocorticotrophic hormone (ACTH) 150 units/m2/day for 3
weeks and then in decreasing dose over 3 to 4 weeks will
often control the seizures, improve the EEG, and
occasionally a child becomes normal (in our experience,
1/10). Some place children on 2 to 4 months of oral
steroids after the ACTH. Others advocate valproic acid
(Depakene) or clonazepam (Klonopin) instead of ACTH,
especially in the symptomatic group where the prognosis is
uniformly unfavorable and the dangerous treatment with
ACTH seems unjustified. In either group oral
anticonvulsants are usually necessary for several years.
It is with this group of children in particular, but also
other children with seizures under the age of 1, that the
pediatrician must avoid polyvalent vaccination, using
instead single vaccines and avoiding pertussis
immunization.

Myoclonic-Akinetic Seizures

Myoclonic seizures are brief jerks (usually
flexor) of an extremity or extremities; if the legs are
involved, the child may be thrown to the ground. Akinetic
spells are a loss of tone rather than a jerk. The spell
may consist only of a head nod or the child may slump to
the floor. These seizures are often part of a mixed
seizure disorder.

Myoclonic-akinetic seizures can be related to
fixed structural lesions, either acquired or developmental
(dysgenesis). However, many degenerative conditions,
especially those associated with widespread grey matter
involvement, have such a pattern. Therefore, the
appearance of these seizures requires a careful search for

degenerative conditions (see Chap. 10). In a significant number of cases, although no recognizable degenerative disorder is present, a deterioration of intellectual performance occurs and eventual psychomotor retardation ensues (Lennox-Gastaut syndrome). In this way a myoclonic-akinetic seizure disorder is similar to infantile spasms. The EEG of this "epileptic encephalopathy" is that of a slow spike wave sometimes called "atypical petit mal." Treatment is difficult despite a broad combination of anticonvulsants. A ketogenic diet (using medium chain triglycerides) is sometimes tried to control the seizures. Valproic acid (Depakene) or clonazepam (Klonopin) may be of particular use in myoclonic-akinetic seizures used singly or in combination with other anticonvulsants. Rarely, steroids can be useful in this group.

Unusual Seizures in Childhood

1. Epilepsia partialis continue is a rare condition characterized by prolonged focal seizures usually without loss of consciousness. Etiologies include chronic focal encephalitis and diffuse cortical or subcortical processes.

2. In benign epilepsy of childhood with a midtemporal spike (Rolandic, Sylvian seizures, or BECRS), seizures are often preceded by a sensory aura around or in the mouth and consist of difficulty speaking, anarthria, facial twitching, and at times drooling. Most commonly they occur just after going to sleep or just prior to waking up. The EEG shows a midtemporal or central (Sylvian, Rolandic) spike focus. These seizures are generally well controlled with phenobarbital, phenytoin, or carbamazepine and the prognosis is excellent in that they are outgrown by puberty. This is an important common subgroup of focal epilepsies.

3. Gelastic seizures are characterized by mirthless laughter. They are seen with focal lesions in the hypothalamus or medial temporal lobe.

4. Reflex seizures are triggered by either photic/visual (most commonly), sensory (proprioceptive), or auditory stimuli that occur unexpectedly.

5. Pseudoseizures are suspected in children who do not respond to anticonvulsants and whose seizures have

atypical features (e.g., prolonged seizures with no postictal period, seizures that consist of "shaking all over," seizures that are never witnessed, seizures with consistently normal EEG patterns). Remember, pseudoseizures may occur in children with known seizure disorders. In children without a seizure disorder who have pseudoseizures, there is usually a role model (family member, friend) whom the child is imitating.

WHAT ETIOLOGIC FACTORS ARE INVOLVED?

Metabolic factors such as hypoglycemia, hypocalcemia, and electrolyte imbalance may play a role at any age. Other "metabolic causes" include uremia, hepatic failure, and hypoxia. Pyridoxine dependency is a cause of neonatal seizures and pyridoxine may help to control seizures secondary to isoniazid (INH) toxicity. Phenothiazines lower the seizure threshold, but are usually safe to use in epileptics if there is an indication and drug levels are adequate.

Exacerbation of a known seizure disorder is common. A child with a controlled seizure disorder who comes to the hospital because of a recurrence often has not been receiving his medication (check blood level), may have outgrown a previous dosage, or has an intercurrent infection. Temporarily increase the medication if seizures occur during a period of intercurrent infection.

//Exacerbation of seizures usually means inadequate medication, noncompliance, or an intercurrent infection.//

Although the late detection of a tumor in children with a longstanding seizure disorder has been reported, if all children with seizures are considered, only rarely is cerebral tumor the etiology.

Warning signs in a child with seizures include: (1) deterioration in school performance; (2) change in the pattern of EEG or seizures; (3) appearance of abnormal signs; and (4) new intracranial calcification. These suggest the possibility of a slow growing tumor or a degenerative disorder. Check blood levels to rule out overmedication as a cause. Re-evaluate completely any child with a well controlled seizure disorder who worsens with no obvious cause.

Post-traumatic epilepsy is most likely to develop during the 1st year after injury; 90% occurs before the end of the 4th year.

Subdural hematoma can be associated with seizures in all age groups (especially infants).

Remember: A seizure is only a symptom of cerebral dysfunction. The clinician must decide whether this symptom represents a fixed, nonprogressive deficit, a progressive intracranial disorder, or idiopathic epilepsy.

LABORATORY AIDS IN DIAGNOSIS

1. Check calcium and glucose levels and perform an EEG in all children with afebrile seizures.

2. Obtain a sleep EEG if a partial complex seizure disorder with temporal lobe origin is suspected and nasopharyngeal leads if necessary.

3. The decision to carry out lumbar puncture (LP) or CAT scan in a child with seizures must be made individually. They are usually performed when there is suspicion of a progressive or focal intracranial disorder. An LP is always done if CNS infection is suspected.

//Treat the child, not the EEG.//

4. Although the EEG is of major importance, the treatment of seizure disorders depends on clinical rather than EEG phenomena. Seizures with a normal EEG, and abnormal EEGs in asymptomatic children are well recognized.

MEDICATION

The major anticonvulsants for focal seizures, major motor seizures (either generalized from onset or those with a focal onset and secondary generalization), and psychomotor seizures are phenobarbital, phenytoin, carbamazepine (Tegretol), primidone (Mysoline), and valproic acid. These drugs are sometimes used together, but a single medication should be increased to maximum doses before adding another.

//Avoid polypharmacy.//

When changing a medication, it is best to make one change at a time (do not eliminate one anticonvulsant until therapeutic levels are reached with the second). In children, phenobarbital is usually the anticonvulsant used first.

For centrencephalic epilepsy with 3 per second spike (absence), ethosuximide (Zarontin) is the drug of choice. Valproic acid (Depakene) may be helpful if ethosuximide is not effective. Valproic acid and clonazepam are useful for seizures associated with atypical spike and wave, e.g., children with akinetic-myoclonic seizures. Methsuximide (Celontin), another medication in the succinimide family, may also be used. Acetazolamide (Diamox) is an excellent adjunct.

Basic Pharmacokinetics

A knowledge of serum half-lives is fundamental to the use of anticonvulsants. It takes 5 half-lives to reach a steady state after each change in dosage, which should be the guide to the timing of the next blood level check.

A. Phenobarbital

1. The average dose is 30 mg twice a day in children (5 mg/kg/day) and 60 mg twice a day in teenagers. The 5 mg/kg/day dose applies only until age 4 or a weight of 20 kg. Older children require approximately 3 mg/kg/day.

2. Therapeutic blood levels are 10 to 50 μg/ml and may vary with the laboratory. (Note units, i.e., μg/ml versus mg/100 ml). Half-life in children and adults is 48 to 96 hours; in neonates, 60 to 160 hours.

3. Phenobarbital may lead to hyperactivity in young children (40%), and an empiric switch to mephobarbital (Mebaral) at 1 1/2 to 2 times the phenobarbital dose is often useful. The elixir tends to cause hyperactivity more than the tablets. Older children and teenagers may not tolerate phenobarbital because of its sedative effects, although the sedative effects often disappear after 10 to 14 days.

4. Phenobarbital is metabolized by the liver and excreted by the kidneys. Levels may increase with concomitant administration of valproic acid (Depakene). Administration of phenobarbital at maintenance doses requires 1 to 3 weeks to achieve equilibrated therapeutic levels.

5. Phenobarbital is available in elixir (20 mg/5 ml) and tablets (15, 30, and 60 mg).

6. Phenobarbital is a very safe, simple, effective, inexpensive drug and therefore is the anticonvulsant of first choice where appropriate in pediatrics.

B. Phenytoin

1. The average dose is 6 mg/kg/day up to 30 kg in children and 200 to 300 mg/day in teenagers. Neonates often require dosages greater than 10 mg/kg intravenously. Absorption by mouth is very poor during the early months of life. Phenytoin can be given in one daily dose in older children if "Kapseals" are used; divided doses in infants and young children may be needed to maintain therapeutic levels when tablets, suspensions, or generic preparations are being used. In our experience the suspension is difficult to use.

2. Therapeutic blood levels are 5 to 20 μg/ml. Half-life in children and adults is 5 to 30 hours; in neonates, 10 to 30; in premature infants, 10 to 140.

3. When phenytoin is administered orally in standard doses it takes 5 to 7 days to achieve therapeutic levels (5 half-lives); intravenous administration in high doses (see section on status epilepticus) gives therapeutic levels immediately. Oral administration in high doses (10 to 15 mg/kg) gives therapeutic levels in 24 to 48 hours. Intramuscular phenytoin may crystallize in muscle and cause muscle damage; it is poorly absorbed. Thus, intramuscular administration should be avoided.

4. Although nystagmus on lateral gaze is a good clinical sign in teenagers that they are taking the medication, it is not present with regularity in young children. Ataxia of gait is a common manifestation of toxicity in all age groups. Phenytoin intoxication may mimic a posterior fossa tumor (nystagmus, ataxia, dysarthria, and diplopia), result in encephalopathy (psychosis), or increase seizure frequency.

5. Phenytoin is metabolized by the liver and regular doses may be given to children who have renal disease or are in renal failure (see valproic acid).

6. A morbilliform rash occurs in approximately 4% of children. If it is important to use the drug, one can stop the medication and restart it slowly. Sometimes

the rash will not recur. Discontinue the medication if the rash persists, as Stevens-Johnson syndrome may occur.

7. Other side effects include hirsutism (no treatment), gum hypertrophy (promote good dental hygiene), and blood dyscrasias secondary to bone marrow toxicity.

8. Isoniazid (INH), diazepam (Valium), methylphenidate (Ritalin), chlordiazepoxide (Librium), and chloramphenicol delay the metabolism of phenytoin and raise plasma levels. Chronic administration of barbiturates may decrease blood phenytoin levels. Children on phenytoin may have factitiously low thyroid function tests. See following section on valproic acid for its interaction with phenytoin.

9. A pseudolymphoma syndrome has been described with phenytoin therapy and usually responds to stopping the medication. Megaloblastic anemia (folate deficiency) and rickets or osteomalacia (low calcium and high alkaline phosphatase) have also been described with phenytoin.

10. An increased incidence of congenital malformations has been reported in infants of mothers exposed to phenytoin during gestation.

11. Phenytoin is available in 100-mg and 30-mg capsules, 50-mg chewable tablets, and suspensions of 6 mg/ml or 25 mg/ml. We recommend only the 6 mg/ml suspension.

//Mistakes in strength of suspension can lead to toxicity.//

C. Carbamazepine (Tegretol)

This drug is becoming increasingly popular because of its lack of side effects, both psychological and cosmetic.

1. Dosage: in children under 8 years of age, 100 mg, 2 to 3 times/day; over 8 years, 100 to 200 mg, 3 to 4 times/day.

2. Therapeutic blood levels are 3 to 12 $\mu g/ml$. Half-life in children and adults is 15 to 30 hours.

3. Toxic side effects include leukopenia, hepatic dysfunction, and rashes. White counts must be checked frequently, as should liver function tests.

4. Erythromycin will elevate Tegretol levels, and thus its use should be monitored carefully.

5. Psychomotor seizures, focal seizures, and occasionally major motor seizures are most likely helped by carbamazepine.

D. Valproic acid (Depakote)

1. Dosage: 15 to 30 mg/kg/day; available in syrup (250 mg/5 ml) or 250-mg capsules. Medication should be administered every 6 to 8 hours to maintain blood levels (more sustained levels are obtained with capsules).

2. Therapeutic blood levels are 50 to 100 $\mu g/ml$. Half-life in children and adults is 6 to 15 hours.

3. Valproic acid is most effective in typical petit mal (absence), myoclonic-akinetic seizures and primary generalized epilepsies. It is unlike any other antiepileptic drug in structure (a short chain branched fatty acid).

4. Valproic acid is a drug with rare hematologic and nephrotoxic side effects. However, there may be significant hepatotoxicity and the medication should be discontinued if monthly liver function tests become significantly altered. There may be transient sedative effects and gastrointestinal disturbances at

onset of therapy, especially if the dosage is built up too rapidly.

5. Interactions with other anticonvulsants include: (a) increased phenobarbital and primidone (Mysoline) levels due to decreased renal excretion (valproic acid causes acidification of urine and thus increased renal tubular resorption of barbiturates); (b) alterations in phenytoin metabolism due to competition for albumin binding sites and changes in liver metabolism may cause increased or decreased serum phenytoin levels. Thus, blood levels of phenobarbital and phenytoin in children receiving valproic acid should be carefully monitored.

E. Clonazepam (Klonopin)

1. The starting dose in children up to age 10 (30 kg) is 0.05 mg/kg/day, and then the medication is increased by 0.25 to 0.5 mg/day to a maximum of 0.2 mg/kg/day in 3 divided doses. In teenagers (60 to 70 kg), starting dose is 1.5 mg/day, increased in 0.5-mg increments/day to a maximum daily dose of 20 mg.

2. Therapeutic blood levels are 5 to 50 μg/ml. Half-life in children and adults is 20 to 40 hours.

3. Clonazepam is used primarily in atypical petit mal, i.e., akinetic-myoclonic epilepsy, and in infantile spasms. It is a member of the benzodiazepine family which includes diazepam (Valium).

4. Drowsiness and ataxia may occur at initiation of therapy, are dose-related, and may be minimized by gradual introduction of medication. Behavioral changes may occur. No serious hematologic or hepatotoxic reactions have been reported, although there are reports of thrombocytopenia.

5. In combination with valproic acid, petit mal status may occur, thus these medications should not be given simultaneously. Do not stop clonazepam suddenly because tonic-clonic status epilepticus may be precipitated (important when one changes from clonazepam to valproic acid).

F. Primidone (Mysoline)

1. Dosage: in children under 8 years of age, 25 to 50 mg, 3 to 4 times/day; over 8 years, 125 to 250 mg, 3 to 4 times/day.

2. Therapeutic blood levels are 4 to 12 μg/ml. Half-life in adults and children is 6 to 18 hours.

3. Primidone must be introduced by small increments to avoid toxicity (oversedation, behavioral disturbances, and gastrointestinal dysfunction).

4. A large portion of primidone is metabolized to phenobarbital (see above); thus, the combination of barbiturates and primidone can lead to oversedation. It is felt that primidone has little to offer over phenobarbital alone. Diazepam plus primidone may also cause oversedation.

   //When testing for primidone (Mysoline) levels, always check phenobarbital levels as well.//

G. Ethosuximide (Zarontin)

1. Dosage: For children 3 to 6 years of age, start with 250 mg/day; for older children, 500 mg/day are usually indicated. The dosage is advanced until a therapeutic level is achieved (40 to 100 mg/ml).

2. The drug is still probably the drug of choice for absence seizures.

3. Toxic side effects include hepatic dysfunction, rashes, eructation and hiccoughs, and leukopenia.

4. Gastric distress is common with dosing, and this may be helped by administering the medicine on a full stomach.

USEFUL ADJUNCT MEDICATIONS

Acetazolamide (Diamox), especially in petit mal and myoclonic seizures, and occasionally in grand mal. It may help prevent seizures associated with menstruation if given a few days prior to the menstrual period.

ACTH for infantile spasms.

<u>Ketogenic</u> <u>diet</u> for difficult to control myoclonic-akinetic seizures.

<u>Blood</u> <u>levels</u> are influenced by compliance (the most common cause of low levels if dosage is adequate), half-lives of drugs, time since last dose, absorption, drug formulations (e.g. "Kapseals," generic drugs), excretion, drug interactions, protein binding, and genetic factors. Toxicity may be influenced by saturable metabolism, i.e., an enzyme limits the rate at which the drug is metabolized. Thus, if the enzyme is overloaded, toxic levels can occur following a minor elevation in dose. This occurs in particular with phenytoin. Therefore, once blood levels are in the therapeutic range, only small increments should be used.

The serum levels of most anticonvulsants can be measured by gas-liquid chromatography. These measurements are important in managing children with poor seizure control and monitoring the reliability of children taking or receiving their medication. Remember, "therapeutic levels" are only a guideline.

Children do not need to remain on anticonvulsants indefinitely. Often they will "outgrow" their seizures. We usually give a child with a normal neurologic examination and normal mentation a trial off medication when he has been seizure free for 3 to 4 years and has no seizure discharges on EEG. Children who have only had a single seizure in the context of illness or are neurologically normal and have normal follow-up EEGs may come off medication in 1 year.

STATUS EPILEPTICUS

Status epilepticus (recurrent convulsions without recovery of consciousness between seizures) is common in children and is potentially dangerous. For status we first use diazepam or lorazepam to stop the seizures, then phenobarbital or phenytoin for continued control. Remember, diazepam may stop seizures, but it does not prevent further seizure activity or stop status epilepticus from beginning again. In addition, diazepam may cause respiratory arrest, especially if the child is on phenobarbital or has received prior doses of barbiturate to control status. In these instances, one must be prepared to intubate the child if diazepam is given. Short acting barbiturates such as amobarbital (sodium amytal) should be avoided because they may cause serious respiratory and cardiac depression. Extensive

experience with intravenous phenytoin in very young
children is not available. We recommend the following
sequence for the treatment of status epilepticus:

1.   Clear airway, oxygen, suction.

2.   Draw blood to check metabolic parameters, especially
     glucose. Check pretreatment blood levels in known
     epileptics.

3.   Start intravenous line, give glucose bolus with 10%
     glucose; maintain blood pressure.

4.   Give diazepam to stop seizures, 1 mg/year of age; a
     maximum of 10 mg for children over 5 years. Diazepam
     is given slowly, 1 to 2 mg i.v./minute in a bolus.
     (It is supplied as 10 mg in 2 ml of buffered solution;
     this may be given via a tuberculin, 1-ml syringe,
     allowing easier administration of 1- to 2-mg doses.)
     Lorazapam is given in doses of 0.05 mg/kg, to a total
     of 2 mg.

5.   Phenobarbital or phenytoin should be given to provide
     continued control or if diazepam is not effective.

a.   Phenobarbital is given 5 mg/kg i.m. in one dose. When
     used as the initial drug in status epilepticus, it may
     be given 1/2 slowly i.v. and 1/2 i.m. or all i.v.
     This i.m./i.v. dose may be repeated in 30 minutes.
b.   Phenytoin is given 10 to 15 mg/kg i.v. over
     approximately 30 minutes. It should not be given
     faster than 25 to 50 mg/minute (1 mg/kg/minute), and
     caution must be used in children with heart disease.
     Maximum dose is 1000 mg. For administration, give by
     slow i.v. push into saline-containing tubing.   If
     given in dextrose and water, it precipitates almost
     immediately. If placed in a burette of saline, a small
     precipitate may develop after 10 to 15 minutes.
     Phenytoin is not absorbed any faster intramuscularly
     than orally; moreover, it may crystallize in muscle.
     It should not be given intramuscularly. After an
     intravenous loading dose, maintenance doses must be
     started.

6.   Paraldehyde is a useful safe medication for status
     epilepticus, especially when other medications prove
     inadequate. The dose is 0.3 ml/kg given rectally
     mixed with an equal volume of mineral oil in a
     nonrubber syringe (not to exceed 5 ml in the child or

10 ml in the teenager). It may be repeated in 1 hour. We do not give paraldehyde intravenously. Paraldehyde should be given with caution in children with pulmonary disease since a major excretion route is through the lungs. (Valproic acid may be given by nasogastric tube or per rectum.)

Prolonged Status Epilepticus

Occasionally seizures are refractory to conventional medications. Check that metabolic parameters are normal (e.g., rule out hyponatremia), that there is no concurrent infection either in the CNS or elsewhere, and that underlying CNS processes are not present, e.g., subdural hematoma, venous thrombosis. Monitor blood levels of anticonvulsants to ensure that adequate levels of medication are present. Steroids and glycerol may be useful if cerebral edema is a complicating factor (see Chap. 22). Rarely, general anesthesia or curare is needed to control seizures that compromise cardiac or respiratory function or cause significant hyperthermia. Remember, more deaths are caused by overtreatment of status epilepticus than by undertreatment.

NOTE: In rare situations surgical treatment of seizures not associated with tumor is possible: (1) intractable temporal lobe seizures, (2) intractable seizures from cortical foci elsewhere, and (3) seizures associated with Sturge-Weber syndrome. It is for the first condition that the greatest experience is available. Such surgery requires an experienced team and the availability of procedures and techniques not ordinarily found outside large referral centers.

TABLE 6.2

NEONATAL SEIZURES AND TIME OF ONSET

	0-3 days	4-7 days	After 10 days
Brain injury	+		
Complicated hypocalcemia	+		
Benign hypocalcemia		+	
Hypoglycemia	+		
Pyridoxine dependency	+	+	+
Infection		+	+
Malformation		+	+
Metabolic defects		+	+
Subdural			+

NEONATAL SEIZURES

Seizures in the neonate (Table 6.2) are not the well organized tonic-clonic movements seen in older children and adults. The movements are frequently multifocal and migratory, although occasionally they are myoclonic or consistently focal. Frequently, there are seizures with only minimal signs such as apnea, eye deviation, or tonic posturing. These may be overlooked unless the baby is observed closely. Do not confuse jitteriness or tremulousness with seizures.

ETIOLOGY

1. Birth Injury: intracranial injury is the major cause of neonatal seizures. This usually takes the form of a hypoxic-ischemic insult, and seizures associated with this encephalopathy occur most commonly on the 1st postnatal day. There may also be cerebral contusions, subarachnoid hemorrhage, and intraventricular hemorrhage. Intraventricular hemorrhage is most common in premature infants (Table 6.3). Seizures associated with birth injury usually occur during the first 3 days of life and sometimes

after the 1st week. Subdural hematomas causing seizures in newborns usually become symptomatic at day 10 or later. Diagnosis of birth injury is based on suggestive history, a bloody spinal fluid, or evidence of subdural hematoma.

2. Metabolic Factors

a. Hypocalcemia (serum level below 7.0 mg/100 ml) occurs during two periods in the neonate. "Early onset" hypocalcemia (days 1 to 3) is frequently associated with causes of perinatal distress such as obstetrical trauma, hypoglycemia, and prematurity; in addition, small-for-dates infants or infants of diabetic mothers are prone to hypocalcemia. At times neonatal hypocalcemia may be associated with maternal hyperparathyroidism or absent parathyroid and thymus glands in the neonate (Di George syndrome). "Late onset" or benign tetany of the newborn occurs on days 4 to 7 and is generally related to the relatively high phosphorus/calcium ratio in cow's milk. This type of hypocalcemia is declining in frequency due to better dietary management and is benign. If seizures are refractory to calcium administration, check magnesium levels.

b. Hypoglycemia is a cause of neonatal seizures in the first 3 days of life (serum glucose below 20 mg/100 ml in the premature and below 30 mg/100 ml in the term infant). Hypoglycemia is seen in small babies, infants of diabetic mothers, and in association with any form of perinatal distress (birth trauma, infection). In these latter situations there may be associated hypocalcemia. Metabolic disorders such as glycogen storage disease and galactosemia may cause persistent hypoglycemia in the newborn.

c. Pyridoxine: pyridoxine dependency is a rare cause of neonatal convulsions. Diagnosis is based on a dramatic response to parenteral pyridoxine.

d. Inborn Errors of Metabolism: maple syrup urine disease, disorders of the urea cycle (hyperammonemia), hyperglycinemia, and propionic acidemia may present in the 1st week of life with seizures. They should be

Table 6.3

SYNDROMES OF INTRACRANIAL HEMORRHAGE IN THE NEWBORN*

Site of hemorrhage	Present-ing day	Fracture	Enlarging head	Sei-zures	Clinical picture	Prognosis	Cerebrospinal fluid	Electro-encephalogram
Intraventricu-lar	1 or 2	Rare	±	+	Infant often premature; se-verely depressed, often flac-cid; bulging fontanelle	Poor	Bloody	Very abnormal (dif-fuse)
Subarach-noid	2 to 10	Rare	−	+	Focal or fragmentary seiz-ures; infant well between seizures; no signs of in-creased intracranial pressure; rarely focal signs	Fairly good	Bloody	May be normal be-tween seizures; focal abnormality
Subdural (he-matoma)	10+	10%	+ (May be asym-metric)	+	Increasing head size often asymmetric, biparietal; brisk deep tendon reflexes, occa-sional focal signs; failure to thrive; lesion may transillumi-nate	Variable; depends on possible asso-ciated cerebral in-volvement	May be clear or xantho-chromatic; rarely bloody	Suppression
Posterior fossa (sub-dural)	10+	Rare	+ (Symmetric)	±	Increasing head size frontally; posterior fossa signs (nystag-mus, decerebration, breath-ing difficulties)	Should be reme-diable surgically	Bloody	Slowing suggestive of increased intracra-nial pressure

* From Bresnan, M. J.: Neurologic Birth Injuries. *Postgrad Med* 49:199, 1971. By permission, McGraw Hill Inc.

suspected if seizures begin after formula feeding in a
baby who was normal at birth and where there is a
family history of unexplained neonatal death.

3. Infection: neonatal seizures secondary to infection
occur between days 4 and 7. Sepsis, bacterial
meningitis, or encephalitis (toxoplasmosis, herpes, or
cytomegalic virus) may be present. Signs of meningeal
irritation are not present in the newborn.

4. Cerebral Malformation: cerebral malformations are
associated with seizures during or after the 1st week
of life.

5. Approximately 25% of seizures in the neonate are of
undetermined etiology. Do not forget maternal
addiction and neonatal withdrawal.

DIAGNOSIS AND TREATMENT

1. Careful antenatal and perinatal history.

2. Check fundi, anterior fontanelle, head circumference,
and transillumination.

3. Lumbar puncture for bleeding or infection.

4. Check metabolic parameters (glucose and calcium) and
administer test infusions.

a. Glucose 50%, 1 to 2 ml/kg i.v. (0.5 to 1 gm/kg).

b . Calcium gluconate 10%: 1 ml (100 mg)/minute, 1 to 2
ml/kg, 100 to 200 mg/kg (EKG monitor); then 5 to 10 ml
p.o. with feeding.

c. Magnesium 0.2 ml (100 mg)/kg of 50% magnesium sulfate
i.v. (30 mg/day p.o.).

d. Pyridoxine 20 to 50 gm i.v.

5. EEG.

6. CAT scan or cranial ultrasound.

7. Anticonvulsants: neonatal seizures rarely compromise
respiration. The drug of choice is phenobarbital 10
mg/kg (1/2 i.v. and 1/2 i.m.) followed by 5 mg/kg/day.
Diazepam (Valium) is given intravenously in a dose of

0.25 to 1.0 mg/kg (do not exceed 2 to 3 mg) but <u>only</u> to stop status epilepticus. Alternatively, Lorazepam may be used (0.05 mg/day). It is dangerous (respiratory and circulatory embarrassment) in infants who have previously received phenobarbital; it affects bilirubin metabolism and may increase the risk of kernicterus. Phenytoin is given in a dose of 6 to 10 mg/kg/day i.v. (it is poorly absorbed intramuscularly and <u>orally</u>).

Remember, do not overtreat. Prognosis is related primarily to the etiology and not to the seizures <u>per se</u>.

PROGNOSIS

Children with paroxysmal, multifocal, or low voltage EEGs have a bad prognosis. Children with normal interictal EEGs or focal EEGs have a better prognosis.

Bad prognostic signs include (1) evidence of CNS disease, e.g., bloody cerebrospinal fluid, meningitis; (2) bulbar palsy requiring tube feeding; (3) apathy, hypotonia, and absent Moro reflex; (4) persistent hemisyndrome; and (5) abnormal eye movements.

FEBRILE SEIZURES

Five to 7% of children will have a seizure during the first 5 years of life, and approximately half of these will be simple febrile seizures. There is a familial incidence of febrile seizures, suggesting an autosomal dominant inheritance with incomplete penetrance.

It is important to distinguish febrile seizures from seizures precipitated by fever. Features of simple febrile seizures are:

1. The age of greatest susceptibility is 9 to 24 months. They are rare under 6 months or after 5 years.

2. The convulsion occurs with the rise of temperature.

3. The fever is usually high, over 39°C (102°F), and there usually is an acute respiratory or ear infection. Roseola and <u>Shigella</u> seem prone to induce febrile seizures.

4. The convulsion is short (15 minutes or less) and generalized; it is predominantly tonic.

5. Seizures do not usually recur in the same infection.

6. Postictally, there is no paralysis or neurologic deficit.

7. An interictal EEG is normal.

8. Recurrence rate: 30% of all children with febrile seizures will have a recurrence. The greatest risk is in children under 1 year of age (50% have a recurrence); the least risk is in children 3 to 5 years old (10% have a recurrence). Fifty percent of recurrences occur within 6 months, 75% within 1 year, and virtually all have occurred within 30 months.

    The following features should make one suspicious that the seizure is not simply febrile in nature.

1. Age: the diagnosis of febrile seizures should not be made in a child under 6 months of age.

2. A prolonged seizure (greater than 15 minutes) with cyanosis.

3. A seizure with a clear focal element.

4. A child known to be febrile for a few days or one with only a slight fever.

5. Repeated seizures during a febrile illness.

6. An abnormal interictal EEG.

    A lumbar puncture on the first febrile convulsion is advisable in most circumstances. This is particularly true in children under the age of 18 months. A focally abnormal EEG implies a significant risk for further seizures and the development of a nonfebrile seizure disorder. The incidence of epilepsy in children with febrile seizures is 2 to 6 times the normal incidence.

    Risk factors for developing epilepsy in children with febrile seizures include:

1. Previously "suspect" neurologic status.

2. "Complex" features of the febrile seizure: duration longer than 15 minutes, more than one seizure in 24 hours, focal features.

3. History of febrile seizures in parents or siblings.

NOTE: Sixty percent of children with febrile seizures do not have risk factors, 34% have one risk factor, 6% have two risk factors. It is this group that appears to warrant prophylactic treatment (see below).

TREATMENT

There is no unanimity of opinion as to when medication should be given for febrile convulsions. It is our practice to recommend prophylactic medication after the second febrile convulsion or after the first seizure if there are indications of a poorer prognosis (see risk factors) or increased risk for recurrence (e.g., young age and positive family history). There is no evidence that oral anticonvulsants given only at the time of a fever are of benefit.

Phenobarbital, 5 mg/kg/day to maintain a therapeutic level of 15 μg/ml, is the drug of choice. Phenytoin does not prevent severe seizures. Medication is always stopped between ages 5 and 6 or after a 30-month period free of seizures if EEGs have been normal. It is likely that briefer periods of treatment (1 year) may be adequate where indicated for many children. While phenobarbital can clearly reduce the incidence of recurrences, there are no data to prove that treatment alters the ultimate outcome.

BREATH-HOLDING SPELLS

Breath-holding spells (peak incidence between 1 and 2 years) are often confused with seizures. A careful history is essential, and parents must be urged to observe the sequence of events. Almost invariably there is a precipitant: trauma, frustration, or another source of pain that causes the child to cry and then hold his breath. There may either be pallor or cyanosis and the child becomes limp. The total episode usually lasts 15 to 30 seconds. Clonic movements may occur with prolonged breath-holding spells as they may in any prolonged syncopal episode. Between spells the EEG is normal.

//Breath-holding spells may
be pallid or cyanotic.//

Studies of children with breath-holding spells have led to them being divided into two categories: pallid and cyanotic. In the cyanotic group prolonged crying and cyanosis precede unconsciousness and there is no change in cardiac rhythm. In the pallid group, there is only a brief cry or "silent" cry, followed by pallor associated with bradycardia and at times asystole. This is a presumed vasovagal episode. The child often becomes rigid and opisthotonic, and the episode is likely to be confused with epilepsy because of the suddenness of the loss of consciousness. Precipitating factors in the cyanotic group are emotionally related (e.g., temper tantrums), while in the pallid group a minor blow to the head or sudden fright is common. In the pallid group there may be a positive family history of syncope, and children in this group may be prone to future syncopal episodes. The prognosis in both types is excellent, with disappearance by age 3 to 4 years. Treatment of the pallid group with tincture of belladonna or Donnatal is often useful. Children who are anemic and have breath-holding spells may improve with correction of the anemia. Anticonvulsants are not helpful in treating breath-holding spells.

BENIGN PAROXYSMAL VERTIGO OF CHILDHOOD

Benign paroxysmal vertigo of childhood is characterized by recurrent attacks of vertigo in children usually less than 5 years of age. There is no loss of consciousness, and the episodes last from a few minutes to several hours. There may be associated vomiting, paleness, and nystagmus. This disorder must be differentiated from a seizure disorder. The EEG is normal and some children later develop migraine. Meclizine may be effective in treating these children.

Suggested Readings

A. Epilepsy

Dodson WE, Prensky AL, DeVivo DC, et al: Management of seizure disorders: selected aspects. J Pediatr 89:527, 695, 1976.
Donohoe NV: Epilepsies of childhood. Postgraduate Pediatrics Series (Apley J edit), Woburn, Butterworths, 1979.
Emerson R, et al: Stopping medication in children with epilepsy. N Engl J Med 304:1125, 1981.
Falkoner MA: Mesial temporal (Ammon's horn) sclerosis as a common cause of epilepsy. Lancet 2:767, 1974.

60

Holmes GL: Diagnosis and Management of Seizures in Children, vol 30 of Major Problems in Clinical Pediatrics. Philadelphia, W.B. Saunders, 1987.

Holowach J, Thurston DL, O'Leary J: Prognosis in childhood epilepsy. N Engl J Med 286:159, 1972.

Lennox WG, Lennox MA: Epilepsy and Related Disorders. Boston, Little, Brown, 1960.

Lerman P, Kivity S: Benign focal epilepsy of childhood. Arch Neurol 32:261, 1975.

Pedley TA (ed.): Pediatric Aspects of Epilepsy. Sixth Annual Merritt Symposium. Epilepsia 28 (Suppl 1): 1987.

Thurston JH, et al: Prognosis in childhood epilepsy: additional follow-up of 148 children 15 to 23 years after withdrawal of anticonvulsant therapy. N Engl J Med 306:831, 1982. (Editorial 306:861).

Tyrer JH: The Treatment of Epilepsy. Current Status of Modern Therapy. Philadelphia, Lippincott, 1980.

B. Drugs

Browne TR: Clonazepam. N Engl J Med 299:812, 1978.

Browne TR: Valproic acid. N Engl J Med 302:661, 1980.

Eadie MJ, Tyrer JH: Anticonvulsant Therapy: Pharmacological Basis and Practice, 2nd ed. London, Churchill Livingstone, 1980.

Glaser GH, Penry JK, Woodbury DM: Antiepileptic Drugs: Mechanisms of Action. New York, Raven Press, 1980.

Hart RG, Easton JD: Carbamazepine and hematological monitoring. Ann Neurol 11:209, 1982.

Penry JK, Newmark ME: The use of antiepileptic drugs. Ann Intern Med 90:207, 1977.

Reynolds EH: Drug treatment of epilepsy. Lancet 111:721, 1978.

Wallace SJ: Carbamazepine in childhood seizures. Dev Med Child Neurol 20:880, 1978.

C. Infantile Spasm

Kurokawa T, et al.: West syndrome and Lennox-Gastaut syndrome: a survey of natural history. Pediatrics 65:81, 1980.

Lacy JR, Penry JK: Infantile Spasms. New York, Raven Press, 1976.

Matsumoto A, et al.: Long-term prognosis after infantile spasms: a statistical study of prognostic factors in 200 cases. Dev Med Child Neurol 23:51, 1981.

Menkes JH: Diagnosis and treatment of minor motor seizures. Pediatr Clin North Am 23:435, 1976.

D. Neonatal Seizures

Volpe J: Neonatal seizures. In Neurology of the Newborn (Volpe J edit), vol. 12 of Major Problems in Clinical Pediatrics. Philadelphia, W.B. Saunders, 1981.

E. Febrile Seizures

Nelson KB, Ellenberg JH: Febrile Seizures. New York, Raven Press, 1981.

F. Breath-holding Spells

Koenigsberger MR, Chutorian AM, Gold AP, Schevy MS: Benign paroxysmal vertigo of childhood. Neurology 20:1108, 1970.
Livingston S: Breath-holding spells in children. JAMA 212:2231, 1970.
Maulsby R, Kellaway P: Transient hypoxic crises in children. In Neurologic and Electroencephalographic Studies in Infancy. New York, Grune and Stratton, 1964.

Chapter 7

Ataxia

Ataxia is a disorder of coordination and rhythm. Because there are many parts of the nervous system that participate in carrying out coordinated movements, ataxia may result from anatomic dysfunction at different levels of the neuraxis. Nevertheless, the various forms of ataxia usually have identifiable clinical features.

ACUTE ATAXIA

Acute cerebellar ataxia of childhood occurs in children between the ages of 1 and 5. The ataxia often follows a febrile illness and develops within hours; it may first be apparent when the child wakes from sleep and is found to be unsteady or totally unable to walk. Gait ataxia is most prominent, although there is some ataxia of the extremities; there may be a generalized decrease in muscle tone and dysarthria. The majority of children recover rapidly, although some are left with mild deficits. The etiology most probably is viral (several types have been isolated from these children including Epstein-Barr virus, i.e., infectious mononucleosis). Cerebellitis is a well recognized complication of chickenpox. The cerebrospinal fluid (CSF) may show a mild lymphocytosis, and there may be nonspecific changes in the EEG. Treatment is symptomatic, and the role of the physician is primarily to rule out other possibilities.

Differential diagnosis includes:

1. Intoxication: intoxication is a common cause of acute ataxia in children, e.g., phenytoin, lead, alcohol,

thallium, or other toxins. Be sure to ask which medicines are in the house.

2. Occult Neuroblastoma: acute cerebellar ataxia may be the presenting feature of occult neuroblastoma. This syndrome includes opsoclonus (irregular, conjugate and dysconjugate, multidirectional, spontaneous eye movements) and myoclonic jerks of the face and body. Any child with cerebellar ataxia plus "opsoclonus-myoclonus" or a nonresolving acute cerebellar ataxia should be screened for neuroblastoma with urinary vanillylmandelic acid (VMA) levels, chest film (mediastinal mass), and plain films of the abdomen or intravenous pyelogram (IVP) (looking for suprarenal calcification). If available, abdominal ultrasound and/or body CAT scan are additional screening options. Some feel the movement disorder represents a remote effect of malignancy on the nervous system.

   "Opsoclonus-myoclonus ataxia" may be seen without neuroblastoma and responds to treatment with ACTH. These children frequently have residual neurologic deficits.

3. Metabolic Disorders: acute intermittent ataxia has been associated with:

a. Maple Syrup Urine Disease (branched chain ketonuria): this condition presents in newborns as seizures; a variant occurs in infants and older children who are otherwise normal apart from attacks of ataxia, irritability, and at times, coma. The attacks are often precipitated by a concomitant infection and diagnosis is suggested by the maple syrup odor of the urine during the attack. There are increased urinary ketones and urinary amino acid analysis shows increased leucine, isoleucine, and valine. Treatment is dietary; some may respond to thiamine.

b. Hartnup's Disease (decreased intestinal absorption of tryptophan and aminoaciduria): these children have intermittent attacks of cerebellar ataxia that may be associated with mental changes, double vision, and a pellagra-like rash (a pruritic rash precipitated by sunlight). Treatment with nicotinamide may be helpful.

c. Pyruvate Decarboxylase Deficiency has been reported in children with intermittent cerebellar ataxia precipitated by fever or excitement. Pyruvate levels may be elevated in CSF, blood, and urine.

d. Arginiosuccinic Aciduria: the most common of the urea cycle abnormalities, may present as ataxia. There is poorly formed hair and frequent mental retardation.

e. Hypothyroidism

4. Acute Intermittent Familial Cerebellar Ataxia: families have been described who have the sudden onset of gait ataxia, intention tremor, and dysarthria. Treatment with acetazolamide may be helpful.

5. Benign Paroxysmal Vertigo of Childhood refers to intermittent attacks of ataxia and vertigo usually lasting minutes. Because the attacks are self-limited, they are not likely to be confused with cerebellar ataxia. The major differential is a seizure disorder or migraine.

6. Guillain-Barre Syndrome or infectious polyneuritis may present as ataxia. Children with Guillain-Barre syndrome are flexic.

7. Posterior Fossa Subdural or Epidural (see Chap. 23)

8. Childhood Multiple Sclerosis, although rare, may be associated with ataxia.

PROGRESSIVE ATAXIA

A. Posterior Fossa Tumors (subtentorial) are common in childhood and often present with ataxia secondary to dysfunction of cerebellum and/or cerebellar pathways. Other cardinal features of posterior fossa tumors are headache, vomiting, papilledema, neck stiffness, and at times head tilt. Other posterior fossa abnormalities may be a cause of chronic ataxia, e.g., Chiari malformation and posterior fossa cyst.

B. Friedreich's Ataxia is a heredofamilial disease occurring in the 1st or 2nd decade. The characteristic features are:

1. Ataxia.

2. Loss of position and vibration sense.

3. Absent deep tendon reflexes.

4. Extensor plantars.

5. Nystagmus and dysarthria.

6. Pes cavus.

7. Kyphoscoliosis. ⟶ *lap problems*

8. Cardiac involvement (EKG abnormalities).

9. Higher incidence of diabetes mellitus.

    The neuropathologic abnormalities are found in dorsal
    columns (position sense), spinocerebellar tracts
    (ataxia), and pyramidal tracts (Babinski response).
    Dorsal root involvement results in loss of reflexes.

C. <u>Ataxia Telangiectasia</u> (Louis-Bar syndrome) is an
    autosomal recessive disease with the following
    features: (1) progressive cerebellar ataxia beginning
    at age 1 to 3; (2) telangiectasia affecting
    conjunctiva and skin (ear) - usually appearing after
    the onset of the ataxia; (3) frequent sinopulmonary
    infections; and (4) decreased reflexes, dysarthria.
    Characteristic laboratory findings include
    immunoglobulin A deficiency, impaired delayed
    hypersensitivity (T cell function), and elevated
    levels of alpha-fetoprotein and carcinoembryonic
    antigen. *B* *Bassen-*

D. <u>Abetalipoproteinemia</u> (Bassen-Kornzweig syndrome):
    this illness begins during the 1st year of life with
    <u>steatorrhea</u>. Later there is progressive ataxia,
    weakness, and retinitis pigmentosa. There are
    acanthocytes (unusually shaped red blood cells) and
    low cholesterol, phospholipid, and triglyceride
    levels. Vitamin E may be helpful.

E. <u>Refsum's Syndrome</u> is due to a deficiency of phytanic
    acid oxidase. It includes ataxia, retinitis
    pigmentosa with night blindness, hypertrophic
    polyneuropathy, deafness, ichthyosis, and cardiac
    conduction defects. CSF protein is elevated and
    phytanic acid is elevated in blood and urine. Dietary
    treatment may be of benefit. An infantile form is now
    recognized.

F. <u>Metachromatic Leukodystrophy</u> often presents with ataxia, both in the childhood and juvenile forms.

G. <u>Hexosaminidase Deficiency</u> (G_{M2} gangliosidosis).

Suggested Readings

Boltshauser E, Deonna TH, Hirt HR: Myoclonic encephalopathy of infants or "dancing eyes syndrome." <u>Helv Paediatr Acta</u> 34:119, 1979.

Gordon N: Intermittent ataxia and biochemical disorders. <u>Dev Med Child Neurol</u> 15:208, 1973.

Kinast M, et al: Cerebellar ataxia, opsoclonus and occult neural crest tumor. <u>Am J Dis Child</u> 134:1057, 1980.

Kinsbourne M: Myoclonic encephalopathy of infants. Symposium on Freidreich's ataxia. <u>Can J Neurol Sci</u> 3:#4, 1976.

Weiss S, Carter S: Course and prognosis of acute cerebellar ataxia in children. <u>Neurology</u> 9:711, 1959.

Acute Hemiplegia

Chapter 8

Acute Hemiplegia

Acute "infantile" hemiplegia or acute hemiplegia of childhood is the sudden development of hemiplegia in a normal child. The tempo of illness is that of a vascular event (stroke), although "infantile hemiplegia" describes a syndrome rather than etiology. Since the advent of cerebral arteriography, the causes of acute hemiplegia of childhood are better understood. In classifying acute hemiplegias, the age of onset and the presence or absence of seizures are important features.

Age of onset is valuable in separating causes of hemiplegia and predicting prognosis. Acute hemiplegias below age 3 years are frequently associated with seizures. Arteriography is usually unremarkable apart from unilateral cerebral swelling. The prognosis is poor with a high incidence of subsequent seizures and mental retardation. Over age 3, seizures at the onset of the hemiparesis and posthemiplegic seizure disorders are less common, vascular occlusion is commonly seen at arteriography, and there is a low incidence of subsequent mental retardation.

Postictal (Todd's) hemiparesis is frequently seen in children after a seizure and does not necessarily represent permanent central nervous system dysfunction or infantile hemiplegia. "Postictal" hemiparesis clears within 24 to 48 hours after cessation of the seizures.

CAUSES OF HEMIPLEGIA

A. Idiopathic

The cause of many infantile hemiplegias is
unknown, especially in children under age 3. They usually
comprise the "hemiplegia-hemiseizure" syndrome; fever and
prolonged seizures often precede the hemiplegia and no
lesion is found at arteriography apart from a swollen
hemisphere. (Some children over age 3 also fall into this
group.) This idiopathic group is listed first as a
"cause" of hemiplegia because of the frequency with which
it occurs.

B. Congenital Heart Disease (CHD)

Cerebrovascular accidents (thromboses) are a well
recognized complication of cyanotic congenital heart
disease, especially in children with polycythemia,
hypoxia, or anemia. The majority of strokes associated
with CHD occur in children under 2. Those with CHD and
right to left shunts are especially prone to develop brain
abscesses, an important differential when a child with CHD
develops hemiplegia.

//Hemiplegia after age 2 years in cyanotic
congenital heart disease is a brain
abscess until proven otherwise.//

However, for reasons not well understood, brain abscess
almost never occurs in children under 2. Brain abscess
may mimic a stroke, but symptoms are usually more
insidious in onset and suggest a mass lesion (headache)
rather than a vascular event. With the advent of early
corrective surgery for CHD, associated neurologic
complications are seen less frequently.

C. Intraoral Trauma

Damage to the carotid artery in the neck or
tonsillar fossa is a well recognized cause of hemiplegia.
A careful history may reveal that the child fell with an
object in his mouth 12 to 24 hours prior to the onset of
the hemiplegia, and an ecchymosis in the posterior pharynx
may be seen on examination. External trauma to the neck
and at times head trauma alone may lead to carotid artery
damage and subsequent hemiplegia.

D. Cardiac Emboli

Cardiac emboli to the brain are associated with the abrupt onset of neurologic signs and symptoms. In children, emboli are most commonly associated with cardiac arrhythmias, cardiac surgery or catheterization, bacterial endocarditis, rheumatic heart disease, or, rarely, cardiac myxoma.

E. Carotid Arteritis

Carotid arteritis is believed by some to be an important cause of childhood hemiplegia. In children with hemiplegia and documented arteriographic abnormalities of the carotid artery, there is a significant incidence of associated ear and throat infection; surgical specimens have shown an arteritis. (Tortuosity, "kinking," and mural dissection of the carotid artery have also been reported in association with childhood hemiplegia.)

F. Systemic Illnesses

Certain systemic illnesses are associated with an increased risk of cerebrovascular disease, including sickle cell anemia, polycythemia, blood dyscrasias, homocystinuria, and polyarteritis nodosa. Children with homocystinuria have an increased incidence of arteriographic complications; if it is suspected, urinary nitroprusside screening for homocystinuria must precede arteriography. Dehydration associated with systemic thrombosis usually involves venous sinuses or superficial veins of the cerebral cortex and can cause seizures that are especially difficult to control. (CSF may have red blood cells as the infarct is often hemorrhagic.)

G. Occlusive Cerebrovascular Disease

Occlusive cerebrovascular disease has been demonstrated arteriographically in children with hemiplegia and no known precipitating or associated factors. Occlusion of large vessels at the base of the brain, lesions of the carotid artery, occlusion of small vessels, and telangiectasia in the basal ganglia have been noted (commonly referred to as "moya-moya" changes). The etiology of these vascular abnormalities is unclear. Some have been related to radiation but are likely due to slow occlusion with development of collaterals.

H. Intracranial Hemorrhage

Intracranial hemorrhage may be associated with hemiplegia, usually in the older child, secondary to hemorrhagic diathesis, e.g., leukemia, angiomatous malformations, and, occasionally, ruptured aneurysm. Trauma, with resultant epidural and/or subdural hemorrhage, may cause hemiplegia and presents certain characteristic features (see Chap. 23).

I. Hemiplegic Migraine

Hemiplegic migraine has been reported in infants and young children. It is a diagnosis that requires exclusion of other processes, e.g., arteriovenous malformation, often by CAT scan or cerebral arteriography. These children have attacks of hemiplegia (sometimes alternating) associated with headache; improvement usually occurs within 24 hours. There is often a family history of migraine. Treatment includes prophylactic phenobarbital or propranolol (see Chap. 13). Ergotamine is contraindicated.

J. Other Rarer Causes

Other rarer causes of acute hemiplegia in children include encephalitis (especially herpes), meningitis with arterial or venous thrombosis, acute hemorrhagic leukoencephalopathy, tumors, and brain abscesses. Stroke-like episodes also occur in the mitochondral encephalomyopathies (MELAS syndrome).

Remember, hemiplegia signifies motor system dysfunction; it does not define the etiology.

PHYSICAL EXAMINATION

General examination should include check of blood pressure, palpation of the carotid arteries, auscultation for bruits (carotid and cranial), careful cardiac evaluation, and examination of the pharynx for intraoral trauma.

Neurologic Examination: in infants and younger children it is usually not possible to precisely localize the lesion responsible for the hemiplegia. Lesions are generally hemispheral, and in the distribution of the middle cerebral artery, the arm is frequently more

affected than the leg. In older children, more precise
localization is usually possible.

Hemiplegia may be secondary to a lesion affecting
the pyramidal tract anywhere from cortex to spinal cord.
Evaluation of associated signs and symptoms, e.g., aphasia
with cortical lesions, determines the level of the lesion.

A. Cortical Lesions: the nature of cortical dysfunction
depends on which hemisphere is involved and the child's
age. Features of cortical lesions common to both
hemispheres include: (1) visual field defect (have child
grasp or identify fingers moved singly and simultaneously
in right and left visual fields); (2) eye deviation (see
Figs. 25.2 and 25.3); (3) pattern of the motor deficit,
e.g., in lesions affecting middle cerebral artery
territory, arm and face are more involved than the leg;
(4) cortical sensory loss: graphesthesia (write numbers
on the palm), stereognosis (identification of an object
placed in the hand).

1. Left Hemisphere: speech function is localized in the
    left hemisphere surrounding the Sylvian fissure in
    almost all right-handed and in two-thirds of left-
    handed children. Aphasia is the hallmark of dominant
    hemisphere lesions; it is a disorder of language
    characterized by difficulty reading, writing,
    comprehending, expressing, and/or naming objects. In
    adolescents, as in adults, if the lesion involves the
    motor cortex, there is decreased speech output and
    associated hemiplegia; comprehension may be spared
    (Broca's aphasia). Lesions posterior to the motor
    cortex give a fluent aphasia, often with difficulty
    comprehending and little or no hemiparesis (Wernicke's
    aphasia). In young children, aphasias are almost
    always nonfluent (child becomes mute or "speechless"
    whether the lesion is anterior or posterior).
    Children generally recover from an aphasia acquired
    before ages 10 to 12, although a high percentage will
    have school problems. If a child can read and write
    without errors he is not aphasic.

2. Right Hemisphere: nondominant hemisphere (parietal
    lobe) function relates to spatial organization and
    body image. Features of right parietal lesions are:
    (a) inattention to the left side. The child may not
    recognize his left hand when it is held in front of
    him and may ignore the left side of a picture; (b)
    constructional apraxia (difficulty copying simple

figures or drawing a clock); and (c) spatial disorganization, e.g., getting lost and confusing directions. The above features of right parietal lesions are not generally seen until teenage years.

B. Brainstem Lesions: the hallmarks of brainstem dysfunction are:

1. Preservation of cortical function, viz., no aphasia or nondominant parietal lobe dysfunction, no field deficit, and no cortical sensory loss or inattention to one side.

2. Crossed hemiplegia, e.g., a right hemiplegia from a left-sided brainstem lesion often produces left-sided brainstem signs, e.g., ataxia or cranial nerve palsy, at the level of the lesion. Thus, a left pontine lesion may produce a right hemiplegia and a left sixth nerve palsy. There also may be crossed sensory signs.

3. Difficulty with eye movements (see Figs. 25.2 and 25.3).

4. Remember, cerebellar signs are common in brain lesions and generally occur ipsilateral to the lesion.

C. Spinal Cord

1. Face is not involved.

2. Hemiparesis is on the same side as the lesion (pyramidal tracts have already crossed).

3. There is often a sensory level, which may be on the opposite side of the lesion (Brown-Sequard syndrome, see Fig. 25.5).

MODE OF ONSET

Emboli usually occur abruptly. The neurologic deficit is maximal at the onset with subsequent improvement; there may be focal seizures.

Thrombosis occasionally occurs abruptly, but often develops in a stepwise or stuttering fashion over hours to days.

Intracranial hemorrhage occurs abruptly, although it may take time before the full deficit develops.

Headache and a stiff neck are usually seen, especially when there is subarachnoid bleeding.

The syndrome of "acute infantile hemiplegia" in children younger than 3 years usually begins with prolonged seizures and fever followed by coma. When the child awakes, the hemiparesis is present. This persists and the child has a recurrent seizure disorder (epilepsy) and is often retarded in development (hemiconvulsion, hemiplegia, epilepsy syndrome-HHE). Despite the clinically suggestive circumstances suggesting a "focal encephalitis," there are no specific laboratory tests.

Remember, hemiparesis present from birth may not be noticed by the family until the child is 3 to 5 months old (e.g., unilateral, persistent fisting or the preferential use of one hand when reaching).

LABORATORY EVALUATION

In addition to routine studies, platelet count, urinary nitroprusside test for homocystinuria, antinuclear antibody, antithrombin III level, protein C, protein S, and sickle cell prep, when appropriate, should be performed. Skull films, EEG, and CAT scan should be done. If the hemiplegia is old and was acquired during the first years of life, skull films may show a unilaterally thickened cranial vault and overdeveloped frontal sinuses (Davidoff-Dyke-Masson abnormality). CAT scan and EEG are almost always positive in cases of supratentorial brain abscess. The CAT scan is very important in the emergency approach to the hemiplegic child as it provides a great deal of information quickly. When done with contrast injection, the ability to identify an arteriovenous malformation, aneurysm, tumor, or abscess is increased. The CAT scan may be normal early in an infarct showing decreased density only after 7 to 10 days. However, it does not give information concerning the dynamic status of blood vessels; therefore, arteriography should be considered early in the course of undiagnosed acute hemiplegia in children. If there is a carotid artery abnormality in the neck, surgical correction is possible. In addition, unsuspected intracranial processes may be revealed, e.g., subdural hematoma or arteriovenous malformation. Lumbar puncture (LP) may provide important data if there is infection or intracranial bleeding. Nevertheless, there is a risk of herniation after LP, especially with brain abscesses and other space-occupying lesions. With fever and hemiparesis, an LP must be done to rule out infection. If a brain abscess or other mass lesion is a possibility, CAT scan or brain scan is indicated prior to LP (see Chap. 19). The physician must decide whether the hemiparesis following seizures might be a Todd's paralysis, not warranting further investigation. Often, 8 to 12 hours of observation will settle the issue.

TREATMENT

Specific treatment depends on the cause of hemiplegia. Control of seizures and maintenance of adequate hydration are very important. Treatment of raised intracranial pressure may be needed (Chap. 22). Physical therapy should be started early, and speech therapy is frequently needed in children with aphasia. Special school help may be necessary.

PROGNOSIS

Although prognosis depends on the underlying cause of the hemiplegia, children younger than 3 years with seizures and hemiplegia have a poorer prognosis and higher incidence of mental retardation and seizures than do hemiplegic children older than 3 years. Children may develop atrophy of the hemiplegic side if the defect is acquired early in life. In addition, posthemiplegia athetosis may occur.

Suggested Readings

Aicardi J, Amsili J, Chevrie J: Acute hemiplegia in infancy and childhood. Dev Med Child Neurol 11:162, 1969.

Byers RK, McLean WT: Etiology and course of certain hemiplegias with aphasia in childhood. Pediatrics 29:376, 1962.

DeVivo DC, Farrell FW: Vertebrobasilar occlusive disease in children. Arch Neurol 26:278, 1972.

Glista GG, Mellinger JF, Rooke ED: Familial hemiplegic migraine. Mayo Clin Proc 50:311, 1975.

Gold AP, Carter S: Acute hemiplegia of infancy and childhood. Pediatr Clin North Am 23:413, 1976.

Gold AP, Challenos YB, Gilles FH, et al: Strokes in children, parts 1 and 2. Stroke 4:833, 1007, 1973.

Isler W: Acute hemiplegias and hemisyndromes in childhood, Clinics in Developmental Medicine. Nos. 41 and 42. Philadelphia, J.B. Lippincott, 1971.

Solomon GE, Hilal SK, Gold AP, et al: Natural history of acute hemiplegia in childhood. Brain 93:107, 1970.

Verret S, Steele JC: Alternating hemiplegia in childhood: a report of eight patients with complicated migraine beginning in infancy. Pediatrics 47:675, 1971.

Chapter 9

Movement Disorders

SYDENHAM'S CHOREA (ST. VITUS' DANCE)

Sydenham's chorea is a movement disorder associated with rheumatic fever that occurs in children most commonly between ages 5 and 15; it is twice as frequent in girls. It may occur prior to, in association with, or after other manifestations of rheumatic fever. It usually occurs as an isolated phenomenon, although approximately one-third of children who present with Sydenham's chorea will develop rheumatic carditis in the future.

//One-third of children with Sydenham's chorea will develop valvular heart disease.//

The clinical picture of a child with Sydenham's chorea is often dramatic:

1. Chorea: involuntary, "jerk-like" movements that may involve fingers, hands, extremities, face, or even the diaphragm. Movements are most pronounced during periods of agitation or activity and are diminished when the child is quiet; they disappear during sleep. The movements often interrupt normal motor activity, and the child may attempt to turn the involuntary movement into a voluntary one. The clinical spectrum ranges from small jerks of fingers to violent chorea that makes the child bedridden.

2. <u>Mental</u> <u>symptoms</u> are common. Prior to the onset of the illness, parents may report emotional disturbances ranging from mild personality changes to psychotic reactions. Children with Sydenham's chorea are usually emotionally labile.

3. The <u>onset</u> of chorea may be abrupt or insidious. At times there may be hemichorea (one-sided) and unilateral weakness.

4. Characteristic <u>physical</u> <u>signs</u> include: (a) generalized hypotonia; (b) "milkmaid grip" (choreic interruption of attempts at maintaining a grip gives the impression of milking a cow); (c) decreased strength; (d) interruption of speech and facial grimacing; (e) inability to maintain the tongue in a protruded position ("Jack-in-the-Box tongue"); and (f) knee reflexes may be pendular; often there is a sustained contraction giving a "hung up" reflex.

DIAGNOSIS AND TREATMENT

The diagnosis is not difficult when there are associated signs, e.g., carditis, a previous history of rheumatic fever, or streptococcal tonsillitis. The child with chorea alone may or may not have elevated acute phase reactants, including antistreptolysin O (ALSO) titer, because there may be a long latent period between the time of the streptococcal infection and the chorea. Cerebrospinal fluid is usually normal; EEG may show diffuse changes. Since one-third of children with chorea will develop rheumatic valvular disease, prophylactic penicillin is recommended until adulthood. Bed rest and sedation are important during the acute stage. Haloperidol may be effective in reducing the chorea. The duration of the chorea is usually 1 to 3 months, and there are generally no or only minimal neurologic sequelae; occasionally the chorea may last longer. Recurrences occur in approximately one-fifth of children. Hyperthyroidism and vasculitis (e.g., lupus erythematosus) affecting the central nervous system may mimic Sydenham's chorea. Persistent hemichorea may be caused by a thalamic glioma. Some studies have suggested that Sydenham's chorea is secondary to autoantibodies directed against basal ganglia nuclei, implying cross-reactivity between the neuronal surface and the streptococcus.

NOTE:

1. An acute idiosyncratic reaction to phenothiazines may cause a dramatic movement disorder (an acute buccolingual dyskinesia occasionally associated with oculogyric crisis) which often responds to intravenous diphenhydramine (Benadryl).

2. <u>Gilles de la Tourette</u> syndrome (<u>tic convulsive</u>) consists of intermittent facial grimacing, multiple tics that may involve the extremities, and vocalizations, including barks and coprolalia (uttering obscenities). Coprolalia is very uncommon before adolescence. Treatment with haloperidol is often helpful. Although previously thought to be of psychiatric origin, Gilles de la Tourette syndrome is now felt to be an organic disturbance, perhaps related to abnormal dopamine metabolism. Its long-term prognosis may not be as bad as originally suspected.

3. A benign chorea may occur in families.

DYSTONIA MUSCULORUM DEFORMANS

Dystonia musculorum deformans is a rare disorder with onset between ages 5 and 15. The fully developed clinical picture is a child twisted upon himself and deformed by the dystonia and permanent secondary contractures. The onset is insidious and often begins with mild dystonic movement of an extremity or the neck, e.g., a foot turned in (plantar flexed), "writer's cramp" (flexion of the hand during writing), or torticollis (neck turned to one side). This slowly progresses to involve the trunk and other extremities. The dystonic postures disappear during sleep unless contractures have developed. Deep tendon reflexes and sensory and cerebellar testing are normal. The initial diagnosis is often psychiatric because of the bizarre positions the children assume. EEG and cerebrospinal fluid studies are normal. Simultaneous electromyograms (EMG) of antagonistic muscles may help in diagnosis. Treatment consists of Valium, L-dopa, and sometimes thalamotomy. Differential diagnosis includes Wilson's disease, Huntington's chorea, and extrapyramidal cerebral palsy.

Suggested Readings

Aron AM, Freeman JM, Carter S: The natural history of Sydenham's chorea. Am J Med 38:83, 1965.

Bird MT, Palkes H, Prensky AL: A follow-up study of Sydenham's chorea. Neurology 26:601, 1976.

Chun RWM, et al: Benign familial chorea with onset in childhood. JAMA 225:1603, 1973.

Eldridge R: The torsion dystonias. Neurology 20:Supplement, 1970.

Erenberg G, et al: The natural history of Tourette syndrome: a follow-up study. Neurology 22:303, 1987.

Golden GS: Tourette syndrome. Am J Dis Child 131:531, 1977.

Nee LE, et al: Gilles de la Tourette syndrome: clinical and family study of 50 cases. Ann Neurol 7:41, 1980.

Chapter 10

Progressive Dementia in Infancy and Childhood

Progressive dementias of childhood encompass a wide spectrum of diseases that result in progressive central nervous system (CNS) deterioration. Most of these diseases are rare and untreatable. Because many are familial, diagnosis is important for genetic counseling. It is impractical for pediatricians to remember all the features of a group of rare diseases that they may never see in practice. In addition, the classification of these entities is not simple. Thus, a basic clinical and laboratory approach to the child with progressive dementia is presented, followed by five diseases selected because they are more common among the progressive dementias or as differentials of common problems, viz., Neimann-Pick disease, Tay-Sachs disease, metachromatic leukodystrophy, Hurler's syndrome, and subacute sclerosing panencephalitis (SSPE). A reference section follows with categorization of progressive dementias according to age of onset (as the problem confronting the clinician is a child with nervous system degeneration beginning at a certain age) and traditional tables of these diseases according to metabolic or anatomic categories.

The clinical approach to a child with possible degenerative disease involves differentiating fixed lesions from progressive defects and ruling out other causes of deterioration.

//Differentiate fixed lesions from progressive ones.//

Loss of intellectual or developmental milestones is the central feature of progressive dementia. Early there is slowing in the rate of new skill acquisition and a failure to achieve milestones at proper times. Actual loss of acquired skills is noticed later but need not be present to make a diagnosis. Other disease processes must be ruled out, e.g., tumor, infection, and hydrocephalus. The diagnosis of a progressive dementia usually will be made on the basis of a suggestive sign (e.g., Hurler-like facies) or a specific metabolic defect (e.g., decreased urine and white blood cell (WBC) arylsulfatase A in metachromatic leukodystrophy).

Establish the following points:

1. Age of onset and rate of progression.

2. Family history.

3. Evidence of grey matter (cortical) dysfunction; early dementia and seizures.

4. Evidence of white matter dysfunction: increased reflexes, upgoing toes, spasticity, and cortical blindness or deafness (seizures occur late).

5. Localized central nervous system dysfunction, e.g., brainstem (nystagmus) or basal ganglia (dystonic) signs.

6. Ocular abnormalities, e.g., cherry red spot, corneal clouding, cataracts, optic atrophy. A cherry red spot is seen in Tay-Sachs disease and in one-half of patients with Neimann-Pick disease and G_{M1}-gangliosidosis; corneal clouding is seen in some mucopolysaccharidoses; cataracts are seen in galactosemia; optic atrophy is seen in the leukodystrophies.

//Careful funduscopic examination is crucial in all children suspected of CNS degenerative disease.//

NOTE: The fundus is a direct anatomic extension of the brain and may mirror the CNS abnormality. Thus, a complete funduscopic examination, through a dilated pupil in a sedated child if necessary, is critical in all children suspected of CNS degenerative disease.

7. Evidence of peripheral neuropathy (decreased deep tendon reflexes, slowed motor nerve conduction times),

e.g., metachromatic leukodystrophy, Krabbe's disease, and neuroaxonal dystrophy.

8. Head size. An enlarged head is seen in Canavan's and Alexander's disease and late in the course of Tay-Sachs disease. (Remember, children with abnormally large heads usually have hydrocephalus or subdural hematoma.)

9. Visceral enlargement, e.g., hepatosplenomegaly, seen in Gaucher's disease, Neimann-Pick disease, Hurler's syndrome, G_{M1}-gangliosidosis, and glycogen storage disease.

10. Skeletal abnormalities, dysmorphic facies (Hurler's syndrome).

Laboratory evaluation includes the following tests when appropriate:

A. Urine

1. Amino acids.

2. Galactose (a positive reducing substance in the urine that is not glucose; Dextrostix negative, Clinitest positive).

3. Dermatan and heparan sulfate (increased in mucopolysaccharidoses).

4. Arylsulfatase A (decreased in metachromatic leukodystrophy).

5. Thiamine triphosphate inhibitor and pyruvate dehydrogenase (Leigh's subacute necrotizing encephalopathy).

6. Copper and ceruloplasmin (altered in Wilson's disease).

B. Serum

1. Amino acids.

2. Hexosaminidase A (decreased in Tay-Sachs disease, G_{M2}-gangliosidoses). Hexosaminidase A and B (decreased in Sandhoff's disease). Alpha-N-acetylglucosaminidase (Sanfilippo syndrome, type B).

3. Glucose and glycogen metabolism (glycogen storage diseases, galactosemia).

4. Uric acid (elevated in Lesch-Nyhan syndrome).

5. Acid phosphatase (increased in Gaucher's disease).

6. Pyruvate and lactate (elevated in Leigh's necrotizing encephalopathy).

7. Measles titer (elevated in SSPE).

8. Ceruloplasmin (low in Wilson's disease).

C. WBC abnormalities include:

1. Arylsulfatase A (decreased in metachromatic leukodystrophy).

2. Beta-galactosidase (decreased in G_{M1}-gangliosidosis), galactocerebroside beta-galactosidase (decreased in Krabbe's disease).

3. Sphingomyelinase (decreased in Neimann-Pick disease), beta-glucosidase (Gaucher's disease), alpha-mannosidase (mannosidosis), alpha-fucosidase (fucosidosis), alpha-iduronidase (Hurler's and Scheie's syndromes).

D. Cerebrospinal Fluid (CSF)

1. Protein (elevated in metachromatic leukodystrophy, Krabbe's disease).

2. Gamma-globulin (marked elevation in SSPE, occasionally elevated in Schilder's disease).

3. Measles titer (elevated in SSPE).

E. Tissue

1. Bone marrow aspirate (characteristic cells are seen in Gaucher's and Neimann-Pick diseases). Foam cells are also seen in G_{M1}-gangliosidosis, Sandhoff's disease, mannosidosis, and fucosidosis. Alder-Reilly bodies are seen in mucopolysaccharidoses.

2. Liver and/or muscle biopsy (glycogen storage disease).

3. Skin and muscle biopsy and electron microscope examination (characteristic abnormalities in many conditions).

PROGRESSIVE DEMENTIAS: FIVE PROTOTYPES

A. Infantile Gaucher's Disease (Type II)

1. Onset 3 to 6 months, death by 1 to 3 years.

2. Clinical

a. Retroflexed head, trismus, and strabismus. (This is a pathognomonic triad.)

b. Hypertonia and dysphagia; later splenomegaly and hepatomegaly develop.

3. Metabolic: glucocerebroside accumulates, pathognomonic Gaucher "reticulum" cell may be seen in the bone marrow, increased acid phosphatase in blood and tissue, deficient leukocyte acid beta-glucosidase.

4. Inheritance: autosomal recessive, no racial predilections.

5. Other: no treatment available, Neimann-Pick disease is one of the major differentials.

B. Tay-Sachs Disease (G_{M2}-Gangliosidosis (Type I)

1. Onset 3 to 6 months. Death by 2 to 5 years.

2. Clinical

a. Loss of milestones is associated with an excessive startle response to noise, light, and touch.

b. After the 1st year of life, seizures (including abnormal laughter, so-called gelastic fits), extensor rigidity, and blindness become prominent.

c. Increased head size may occur, usually after 15 months of age.

d. Almost all children have a cherry red spot by 6 months.

3. Metabolic: decreased serum hexosaminidase A.

4. Inheritance: autosomal recessive; most carriers are Jewish and can be identified; prenatal diagnosis is possible. Sporadic cases occur in the non-Jewish population.

5. Other: in some communities, screening programs for the Jewish population are available to identify couples who may both be carriers. One in 27 Ashkenazi Jews are carriers and approximately 50 new cases of the Tay-Sachs disease occur in the United States each year.

6. NOTE: Sandhoff's disease is phenotypically similar to Tay-Sachs disease, but is not associated with the Jewish population. Hexosaminidase A and B are both deficient.

C. Infantile Metachromatic Leukodystrophy (Sulfatide Lipidosis)

1. Onset 15 to 18 months. Death by 5 to 8 years.

2. Clinical

a. The disorder usually begins as a gait disturbance (ataxia) in the toddler; within a year there are bulbar signs, hypotonia followed by spasticity, and intellectual deterioration.

b. Later, loss of speech, optic atrophy associated with a grayish macular change, and decerebrate posturing.

c. A clinical hallmark during the initial stages is loss of reflexes secondary to an associated peripheral neuropathy in the presence of spasticity.

d. Seizures may occur but are not prominent; there may be absent gallbaldder function.

3. Metabolic: decreased urinary or WBC aryl sulfatase A activity; CSF protein is elevated.

4. Inheritance: autosomal recessive, diagnosis may be made in utero.

D. Hurler's Syndrome (Gargoylism: Mucopolysaccharidosis Type IH)

1. Onset: toward the end of the 1st year of life it becomes apparent that the child is retarded in development and has an abnormally shaped head.

2. Clinical

a. As the child grows, the characteristic features of gargoylism become apparent: characteristic facies, a dwarfed stature, joint contractures, gibbus, a protuberant abdomen (hepatosplenomegaly), short stubby hands, valvular heart disease, deafness, and corneal clouding (present since birth).

b. Some children may develop communicating hydrocephalus secondary to leptomeningeal thickening and subarachnoid cysts.

c. Death occurs by age 10 to 20 years.

3. Metabolic: there is a deficiency of alpha-iduronidase, and abnormal amounts of heparan and dermatan sulfate are excreted in the urine; metachromatic cytoplasmic inclusions may be found in peripheral leukocytes and bone marrow cells.

4. Inheritance: autosomal recessive and diagnosis may be made in utero.

E. Subacute Sclerosing Panencephalitis (SSPE, Dawson's Encephalitis)

1. Onset 5 to 15 years of age with death 3 to 7 years later.

2. Clinical

a. Initial symptoms are usually subtle and consist of personality changes and poor school performance).

b. Later, characteristic "slow" myoclonic jerks involving limbs or trunk and then progressive neurologic deterioration leading to a state of unresponsiveness.

c. Characteristic EEG abnormalities (paroxysmal high voltage slow waves with a "burst-suppression" pattern) parallel the myoclonic jerks. Diazepam may bring out EEG abnormalities early in the course.

3. Metabolic: SSPE is related to a preceding measles infection (virus has been cultured from brains of children with SSPE), and children have increased measles titers in blood and CSF in addition to a markedly elevated CSF gamma-globulin. In the brain, there are neuronal inclusion bodies that are composed of paramyxovirus-like particles.

4. Other: treatment with gamma-globulin and antiviral agents has not been successful. Most of these children come from rural rather than urban environments and their measles infection often occurred at an early age (under age 2).

PROGRESSIVE DEMENTIAS CATEGORIZED ACCORDING TO AGE OF ONSET (The following age categories represent a general classification and are not meant to be exclusive.)

Onset at Birth

A. (Generalized) G_{M1} Type I Gangliosidosis

1. Clinical

a. Infants have coarsened facial features with hirsutism, nonpitting edema of limbs, heptosplenomegaly, and kyphoscoliosis.

b. Late in the 1st year, they progress to a state of decerebrate rigidity with an exaggerated startle response to sound and seizures.

c. One-half have a cherry red spot.

d. Death by age 2.

2. Metabolic: lipid-laden histiocytes are found in liver, spleen, and bone marrow; beta-galactosidases A, B, and C are nearly absent.

3. Inheritance: autosomal recessive; prenatal diagnosis is possible.

B. Alexander's Disease

1. Clinical

a. Progressive enlargement of the head which begins at birth.

b. Muscular weakness, contractures, and retardation.

c. Death by age 1 to 2.

2. Metabolic: Rosenthal fibers (fibrinoid bodies deposited extracellularly) disrupting myelin are the pathologic landmark. Premorbid laboratory diagnosis is not possible.

C. Type I (von Gierke's) Glycogen Storage Disease

1. Clinical

a. Seizures and hepatomegaly with metabolic acidosis and hypoglycemia.

b. Neurologic abnormalities relate to the severity of the hypoglycemia.

c. Survival is possible if metabolic abnormalities are corrected by constant feeding, usually via gastrostomy.

2. Metabolic: glucose 6-phosphatase is deficient, and blood glucose levels do not respond to glucagon or epinephrine.

3. Other: treatment is with exogenous glucose.

D. T Cell Disease (mucolipidosis II)

Onset: 1 to 3 weeks

A. Maple Syrup Urine Disease

1. Clinical

a. Normal at birth; progressive cerebral deterioration begins a fews days after the first protein feeding with seizures, lethargy, vomiting, and increased muscle tone.

b. There may or may not be a maple syrup odor of the urine.

c. Death by 1 year.

2. Metabolic: inborn error of the metabolism of branched chain amino acids producing increased urinary ketones, leucine, isoleucine, and valine; there may be hypoglycemia.

3. Inheritance: autosomal recessive.

4. Other: dietary treatment is possible; some respond to thiamine. (An intermittent form occurs in older otherwise normal children which is precipitated by other illnesses and is manifested as stupor, irritability, and ataxia (see Chap. 7).)

B. Galactosemia

1. Clinical

a. Diarrhea and vomiting begin with mild feeding; later there is hepatic (jaundice) and renal dysfunction (proteinuria and aminoaciduria).

b. Seizures and cataracts usually develop at 1 to 2 months.

c. Death or severe retardation occurs by age 1 to 2 if not treated.

2. Metabolic: ingested galactose (from milk) accumulates due to a deficiency of galactose 1-phosphate uridyl transferase or galactose kinase. There is generalized aminoaciduria and a positive reducing substance in the urine that is not glucose. It will give a positive Clinitest but a negative Dipstix (the former only measures reducing substance; the latter measures glucose).

3. Inheritance: autosomal recessive; heterozygotes may be identified.

4. Other: removal of dietary galactose is effective treatment.

Onset: 1 to 3 Months

A. Type II (Pompe's) Glycogen Storage Disease

1. Clinical

a. After a brief period of normal development, progressive hypotonia and muscle weakness associated with cardiomegaly, hepatomegaly, and an enlarged tongue develop.

b. Since glycogen is also deposited in the motor nuclei of brainstem and spinal cord, there is swallowing difficulty and, later, absent reflexes.

c. Death by 1 year.

2. Metabolic: absent acid maltase (alpha-1,4-glucosidase) leads to glycogen accumulation.

3. Inheritance: autosomal recessive.

4. Other: a late onset form presents as a pure myopathy of the limb-girdle type.

B. Haltia-Santavuori variant of neuronal ceroid-ceroid-lipofuscinosis

Onset: 3 to 6 Months

A. Gaucher's Disease: (see p. 84)

B. Tay-Sachs Disease: (see p. 84)

C. Krabbe's Disease (Globoid Leukodystrophy)

1. Clinical

a. Progressive spasticity, rigidity, tonic spasms, and nystagmus; there may be optic atrophy.

b. Peripheral neuropathy (may be detectable only by nerve conduction).

c. Death by 2 to 3 years.

2. Metabolic: a deficiency of galactocerebroside beta-galactosidase can be identified in WBCs and is associated with a characteristic globoid cell reaction of the white matter; there is elevation of CSF protein.

3. Inheritance: autosomal recessive; in utero diagnosis is possible.

D. Neimann-Pick Disease (Type A)

1. Clinical

a. Massive hepatosplenomegaly associated with progressive spasticity, blindness, and psychomotor retardation.

b. Often a history of neonatal jaundice, there may be a cherry red spot.

c. Death by 1 to 4 years.

2. Metabolic: sphingomyelin accumulates, diagnosis is made by finding characteristic foam cells on liver or bone marrow biopsy and sphingomyelinase deficiency in white cells.

3. Inheritance: autosomal recessive; many affected infants are Jewish.

4. Other: type B is seen at ages 1 to 4 and consists only of visceral enlargement; types C and D involve the CNS subacutely, occur between ages 2 and 10 years, and have only minimal hepatosplenomegaly.

E. Phenylketonuria (PKU)

1. Clinical

a. A normal child at birth; a severely defective child at 1 year if untreated.

b. Agitated behavior, hypertonia, increased reflexes, hyperkinesia, tremor seizures, EEG abnormalities, atopic eczema, microcephaly, and in over one-half of the children, a fair complexion.

c. Occasionally patients with PKU may have normal intelligence.

2. Metabolic: absence of phenylalanine hydroxylase, associated with defective myelin and brain protein formation. Diagnosis is via urine and serum amino acid pattern.

3. Inheritance: autosomal recessive; heterozygotes usually can be identified.

4. Other: Dietary treatment is effective. Atypical cases resembling PKU but not responding to dietary manipulation are being recognized. One variant associated with severe seizures in early infancy has been identified with a deficiency in tetrahydrobiopterin reductase and is not ameliorated by a low phenylalanine diet.

F. Multiple Amino Acid Deficits

1. There are several amino acid deficits associated with progressive psychomotor retardation and seizures in the first year of life, e.g., hypersarcosinemia, hyperbeta-alaninemia. They are screened for by urine and serum amino acid testing.

G. Canavan's Disease (Spongy Degeneration of White Matter)

1. Clinical

a. Marked early increase in head size (a characteristic feature) often with splitting of the sutures.

b. Hypotonia followed by spasticity, progressive psychomotor retardation, and blindness.

c. Death by 2 years.

2. Metabolic: no known abnormality; diagnosis is made by brain biopsy or at autopsy with the pathologic feature being spongy degeneration of the white matter.

3. Inheritance: incidence is higher in Jewish infants.

Onset: 3 to 12 Months

A. Lesch-Nyhan Syndrome (Hyperuricemia, Athetosis, and Self-Mutilation)

1. Clinical

a. Delayed motor development at 3 to 4 months, extrapyramidal signs at 8 to 12 months.

b. At 2 to 3 years, self-mutilation, with biting of fingers, lips, and buccal mucosa.

c. Many children have seizures.

2. Metabolic: uric acid is elevated due to a deficiency of hypoxanthine-guanine phosphoribosyl transferase (there may be renal stones).

3. Inheritance: sex-linked; heterozygotes can be identified.

4. Other: treatment does not help CNS dysfunction and no characteristic pathologic changes are noted at autopsy.

B. Pelizaeus-Merzbacher Disease

1. Clinical

a. Oscillating, wheeling nystagmus that appears during the 1st year.

b. Spasticity, ataxia, intention tremor, choreoathetosis, Parkinsonian features, and intellectual deterioration occur over years.

c. May be mistaken for Leigh's encephalopathy (see p. 95).

2. Metabolic: No known abnormalities; diffuse dymelination with a tendency to spare perivascular islands of myelin is seen at autopsy.

3. Inheritance: sex-linked.

Onset: 6 Months to 2 Years

A. Juvenile G_{M1} Gangliosidosis Type II

1. Clinical

a. Ataxia, strabismus, muscle weakness, progressive spasticity, and psychomotor retardation.

b. Some of the children have characteristic radiologic findings consisting of beaking of lumbar vertebrae and pointing of the metacarpal bones; there is no ocular or visceral involvement.

c. Death by 3 to 10 years.

2. Metabolic: beta-galactosidase deficiency; heterozygotes can be identified by examination of

white blood cells or cultured skin fibroblasts; prenatal diagnosis is possible.

3. Inheritance: autosomal recessive.

Onset: 6 Months to 4 Years

A. Homocystinuria

1. Clinical

a. Shuffling gait, malar flush, livedo reticularis, fine hair, fragile skin, ectopic lenses, and seizures.

b. One-half of children are mildly to severely retarded.

c. A marked tendency to develop thromboembolic phenomena involving major vessels; prone to complications from cerebral arteriography.

d. Resemble patients with Marfan's syndrome (tall, long extremities).

2. Metabolic: liver cystathionine synthetase is deficient and diagnosis is based on urine examination for amino acids (or nitroprusside screening); treatment is dietary and vitamin B6.

3. Inheritance: autosomal recessive.

Onset: 1 to 3 Years

A. Hurler's Syndrome (see p. 86).

B Metachromatic Leukodystrophy (see p. 100).

C. Neuroaxonal Dystrophy

1. Clinical

a. Psychomotor retardation, spasticity, optic atrophy, and often nystagmus.

b. There may be a neuropathy with lack of movement and loss of pain sensation in the lower extremities.

c. Death by 6 to 10 years.

2. Metabolic: no known defect.

3. Other: diagnosis is made at autopsy although the sensory loss may be marked and generalized, suggesting the diagnosis during life.

D. Leigh's Necrotizing Encephalomyelopathy

1. Clinical

a. Eye signs: nystagmus, jerky eye movements, and pupillary abnormalities.

b. Hypotonia, ataxia, and progressive psychomotor retardation.

c. Weakness, anorexia, and respiratory difficulties; some have marked tachycardia.

d. Death 1 to 3 years from onset.

2. Metabolic: abnormally high blood pyruvate and lactate levels and a thiamine triphosphate inhibitor in the urine.

3. Other: pathologically, the disease is similar to Wernicke's encephalopathy seen in adults, except the mamillary bodies are spared. Treatment with massive doses of thiamine has not been very successful; spontaneous remissions may occur.

Onset: 1 to 6 Years

A. Type C Neimann-Pick Disease

1. Clinical

a. Children are normal until after age 2 when they develop mild spasticity, a slowly progressive dementia, seizures, and mild hepatosplenomegaly.

b. There may be a cherry red spot.

c. Death late in the first decade.

2. Metabolic: membrane-bound sphingomyelinase is deficient, sphingomyelin and cholesterol are increased in the viscera, and total sphingomyelinase activity is normal; characteristic foam cells may be seen on bone marrow.

Onset: <u>2</u> <u>to</u> 5 <u>Years</u>

A. <u>Late Infantile Amaurotic Idiocy Form of Neuronal</u>
<u>Ceroid Lipofuscinosis</u> (Jansky-<u>Bielschowsky Disease</u>,
<u>Batten's Disease</u>)

1. Clinical

a. Myoclonic seizures, retardation, and then optic
atrophy with progressive visual loss. There is a
characteristic retinal granular macular degeneration.

b. Death by age 2 to 8 years.

2. Metabolic: unlike the gangliosidoses, this form of
amaurotic idiocy has no known chemical abnormality;
ganglion cells appear swollen with a lipofuscin-like
material.

3. Inheritance: there is no racial predilection.

4. Other: diagnosis is made clincally and by electron
microscopic examination of skin.

Onset: <u>2 to 6 Years</u>

A. <u>Hunter's Syndrome</u>: <u>Mucopolysaccharidosis</u> (<u>MPS</u>) <u>Type</u>
<u>II</u>

1. Clinical

a. A milder form of MPS (to be distinguished from
Hurler's syndrome) with less mental retardation, no
corneal opacities, and a later onset.

b. Characteristic facies, hepatosplenomegaly, and
skeletal deformities with abnormal posture, dwarfism,
and early deafness. White spots on the back between
the scapulae are characteristic.

c. Children live into adulthood.

2. Metabolic: defect in iduronosulfate sulfatase;
abnormal amounts of heparan sulfate and dermatan
sulfate in the urine.

3. Inheritance: sex-linked; diagnosis may be made <u>in</u>
<u>utero</u>.

B. G_{M2} Type III Gangliosidosis (Juvenile)

1. Clinical

a. Ataxia, loss of speech, progressive spasticity, and athetoid posturing.

b. There is optic atrophy and sometimes a cherry red spot; loss of vision occurs late.

c. Death by age 5 to 15 years.

2. Metabolic: a partial deficiency of hexosaminidase A.

3. Inheritance: autosomal recessive; prenatal diagnosis and identification of heterozygotes are possible.

Onset: 4 to 8 Years

A. Juvenile Amaurotic Idiocy Form of Neuronal Ceroid Lipofuscinosis (Spielmeyer-Sjogren's Disease)

1. Clinical

a. Visual failure is the first symptom, followed by seizures and then psychomotor retardation.

b. Difficulty walking, spasticity, dystonia, rigidity, and akinesia.

c. The fundus shows a pale macula surrounded by dark brown spots. Some patients have no retinal abnormality.

d. Death in the second decade.

2. Metabolic: none known, see Jansky-Bielschowsky disease (p.).

3. Other: an adult form of neuronal ceroid lipofuscinosis, Kufs' disease, has also been described.

B. Sanfilippo Syndrome: Mucopolysaccharidosis Type III

1. Clinical

a. Severe mental retardation; there may be associated seizures and athetosis.

b. Mild hepatosplenomegaly and minimal, if any, corneal clouding.

c. Few of the clinical x-ray features seen in Hurler-Hunter patients.

2. Metabolic: there are three metabolic varieties of Sanfilippo syndrome. In type A, the defect is heparan-N-sulfamadase; in type B, N-acetyl-alpha-glucosaminidase. In type C, heparin N-acetylglucosamine transferase is deficient. There is excess excretion of heparan sulfate in the urine.

3. Inheritance: autosomal recessive.

4. Other: mucopolysaccharidosis IS, IV, and VI, (Sheie's, Morquio's, and Maroteaux-Lamy syndromes) have mild or no mental retardation; there are skeletal changes and corneal clouding.

Onset: 5 to 10 Years

A. Schilder's disease

Schilder's Disease actually includes two entities: one form (sporadic), probably is the equivalent of juvenile multiple sclerosis; the other is sex-linked adrenoleukodystrophy. Their clinical presentation may be identical.

1. Clinical

a. A progressive form manifested by neuropsychological difficulties, pyramidal tract signs, cortical blindness (fundus is normal and pupillary reflex is intact), and deafness.

b. A pseudotumor form with papilledema and symptoms of raised intracranial pressure.

c. A predominantly psychiatric form with no focal neurologic signs.

d. A polysclerotic form similar to multiple sclerosis with discrete episodes of neurologic dysfunction.

2. Metabolic: in the sex-linked adrenoleukodystrophy, the ratio of C22/26 fatty acids in cultured skin fibroblasts is abnormal.

3. Inheritance: a specific sex-linked form exists that is associated with adrenal insufficiency and skin pigmentation (adrenoleukodystrophy, bronze Schilder's disease). Treatment with steroids in these cases is of no benefit apart from helping the adrenal insufficiency; there is no specific pattern of inheritance in other forms.

4. Other: gamma-globulin may be elevated in the CSF. Pathologically, there is demyelination of large areas of white matter in the cerebral hemispheres, especially occipitally. In the sporadic variety the pathologic process is similar to multiple sclerosis and may represent a childhood variant.

B. Huntington's Chorea

1. Clinical

   In children there may be a Parkinsonian-like picture (bradykinesia, loss of associative movements, and rigidity) or chorea and dystonia.

b. Convulsions and progressive dementia occur in both children and adults, though convulsions are rare in adults.

c. Death may occur 5 to 10 years after onset.

2. Metabolic: glutamic acid decarboxylase deficiency in basal ganglia, although this is probably a secondary change.

3. Inheritance: autosomal dominant; thus, there is a positive family history (more common on the male side, i.e., the father is most often the affected carrier).

4. Other: EEG is abnormal with spike discharges. CAT scan or MRI shows atrophy of the caudate nucleus with normal temporal horns. There is no treatment for the dementia; the chorea may be helped by haloperidol (Haldol) or tetrabenazine.

Onset: <u>8</u> <u>to</u> <u>15</u> Years

A. <u>Myoclonic</u> <u>Epilepsy</u> (<u>Lafora</u> <u>Body</u> <u>Disease</u>)

1. Clinical

a. Generalized seizures, myoclonus, gait difficulties, and progressive intellectual deterioration.

b. EEG is markedly abnormal with multiple spikes; CSF is normal.

c. Death 5 to 20 years after onset.

2. Metabolic: none known. Pathologically there are neuronal inclusion (Lafora) bodies and inclusions can be found in other tissues as well, especially liver and muscle.

3. Inheritance: autosomal recessive; there is no treatment apart from seizure control with anticonvulsants.

Onset: <u>10</u> <u>to</u> <u>12</u> Years

A. <u>Type</u> <u>D</u> <u>Neimann–Pick</u> <u>Disease</u>

1. Clinical: this slowly progressive degenerative disease (hepatosplenomegaly, seizures, and intellectual deterioration) has been described in Catholics from Nova Scotia. Death occurs within 10 to 15 years.

Onset: <u>5</u> <u>to</u> <u>20</u> Years

A. <u>Juvenile</u> <u>Metachromatic</u> <u>Leukodystrophy</u>

1. Clinical features are similar to the late infantile form (p. 85).

a. A previously normal child develops a gait disturbance, spasticity with a peripheral neuropathy, and then begins a downhill course that includes progressive intellectual impairment, loss of speech, and decerebrate posturing.

2. Other: laboratory diagnosis and inheritance are the same as in the infantile form. (An adult form has

also been described presenting as a psychiatric
disorder.)

B. Hallervorden–Spatz Syndrome (Pigmentary Degeneration
of the Globus Pallidus

1. Clinical

a. Gait difficulties, with extrapyramidal dysfunction
(athetosis, dystonia, and rigidity), progressive
dementia, convulsions, and at times, spasticity.

b. Death by 5 to 15 years after onset.

2. Metabolic: none known.

3. Inheritance: no specific pattern.

4. Other: pathologically there is brown pigmentation
(iron) in the globus pallidus and substantia nigra.
Treatment has included iron chelation, L–dopa, and
amantadine. The major differential diagnoses are
Wilson's disease and childhood Huntington's chorea.

C. Wilson's Disease (Hepatolenticular Degeneration)

1. Clinical

a. Basal ganglia signs (dystonia, tremor, and chorea), a
Kayser–Fleischer ring, and liver dysfunction (liver
failure mimicking hepatitis often is the presenting
sign of Wilson's disease in children).

b. May present as a psychiatric disorder or seizures plus
dementia.

2. Metabolic: an inborn error of copper metabolism,
associated with low serum ceruloplasmin and an
elevated urinary copper; there may be aminoaciduria.

3. Inheritance: autosomal recessive. Siblings of
children with Wilson's disease should be screened.
They may be asymptomatic yet affected and warrant
prophylactic treatment.

4. Other: treatment with penicillamine and other
chelators is effective; it is important to screen
patients with evidence of basal ganglia dysfunction or
chronic hepatitis for Wilson's disease.

D. Gaucher's Disease Type III (Juvenile)

E. Mucolipidosis I (cherry red spot, myoclonus, epilepsy variant).

TABLE 10.1

DISEASES OF WHITE MATTER

Disease	Onset
Alexander's disease (hyaline pancephalopathy)	At birth
Canavan's disease (spongy degeneration of the white matter)	3-6 months
Krabbe's globoid cell leukodystrophy	3-6 months
Pelizaeus-Merzbacher disease	3-12 months
Metachromatic leukodystrophy	1-2 years
Schilder's disease	5-10 years
SSPE	5-15 years

Table 10.2

MUCOPOLYSACCHARIDOSES

Type	Skeletal changes	Enzyme deficit	Mental retardation	Hepatosplenomegaly	Corneal clouding	Onset course	Urine excretion
IH Hurler	Marked	Alpha-L-Iduronidase	Severe	Marked	Severe	1st year progressive	Dermatan SO_4 Heparan SO_4
IS Scheie	Mild	Alpha-L-Iduronidase	Mild—none	Variable	Severe	5-10 years; intermediate course, aortic disease	Dermatan SO_4 Heparan SO_4
II Hunter (A milder form also exists)	Marked	Iduronosulfate sulfatase	Severe (gradual onset)	Moderate	None	2-5 years; milder than Hurler's	Dermatan SO_4 Heparan SO_4
III Sanfilippo	Mild	Heparan-N-sulfamidase (Type A); N-acetyl-alpha-glucosaminidase (Type B)	Severe	Slight	None	5-7 years; mild course	Heparan SO_4
IV Morquio	Marked	N-acetylhexosamine sulfate sulfatase	Mild—none	Slight	None	1-2 years; intermediate course, aortic disease	Keratan SO_4
VI Maroteaux-Lamy (A milder form also exists)	Marked	Arylsulfatase B	None	Moderate	Moderate	2-3 years	Dermatan SO_4
VII Beta-Glucuronidase deficiency	Moderate	Beta-glucuronidase	Moderate	Moderate	None	2-4 years	Dermatan SO_4

TABLE 10.3

GANGLIOSIDOSES

Name	Onset
G_{M2} type I (Tay-Sachs)	3-6 months
G_{M2} type II (Sandhoff's)	3-6 months
G_{M2} type III ("juvenile" Tay-Sachs)	2-6 years
G_{M1} type I (generalized gangliosidosis)	At birth
G_{M1} type II (juvenile)	6 months - 2 years

TABLE 10.4

NEIMAN-PICK AND GAUCHER'S DISEASES

Name	Onset
Gaucher's type I	Adult onset
Gaucher's type II (infantile)	3-6 months
Gaucher's type III (juvenile)	10-20 years
Neimann-Pick Type A	3-6 months
Type B	5-10 years
Type C	2 years, 1st decade
Type D	8-12 years

TABLE 10.5

NEURONAL CEROID LIPOFUSCINOSES

Type	Onset
Haltia-Santavuori variant	1-3 months
Late infantile amaurotic idiocy (Jansky-Bielschowsky, Batten)	1-4 years
Juvenile amaurotic idiocy (Spielmeyer-Sjogren)	Onset 4-8 years, death in 2nd decade
Adult form (Kufs')	20's

TABLE 10.6

GLYCOGEN STORAGE DISEASES

(These diseases may present as myopathies, retardation, or hypoglycemia with seizures.)

Type – name	Onset and course
I von Gierke's	Infancy; survival if treated
II Pompe's	1–3 months, death by 1 year
II Late infantile acid maltase deficiency	Childhood, survival
III Cori's	1–3 months, survival
IV Andersen's	1–6 months, death at 1 year (longer survival with proper diet)
V McArdle's	Childhood, survival
VI Hers'	Childhood, survival
VII Tauri's	Childhood, survival

TABLE 10.6 (cont.)

GLYCOGEN STORAGE DISEASES

Enzyme deficiency	Features
I Glucose 6-phosphatase	Neonatal seizures, hepatomegaly and hypoglycemia.
II Acid maltase	Hypotonia, cardiomegaly, hepatomegaly and macroglossia. Swallowing difficulty.
II Acid maltase	Slowly progressive weakness (myopathic). Cardiac or visceral enlargement.
III Debrancher	Hypoglycemia, hepatomegaly, and hypotonia.
IV Brancher	Failure to thrive, hepatosplenomegaly.
V Muscle phosphorylase	Cramping after exercise.
VI Liver phosphorylase	Growth retardation, hypoglycemia, and hepatomegaly.
VII Phosphofructokinase	Cramping and fatigue after exercise.

(Isolated cases of other glycogen storage diseases secondary to other enzyme deficiencies and associated with weakness, hypoglycemia, or retardation have also been reported.)

TABLE 10.7

DISORDERS OF AMINO ACIDS

Type	Onset
Phenylketonuria	1st year
Maple syrup urine disease	Infancy, childhood
Homocystinuria	Early childhood
Hartnup's disease	Early childhood

(There are case reports of several varieties of amino acid disorders (e.g., hypersarcosinemia and hyperbeta-alaninemia) often associated with seizures and retardation.)

An alternative organizational approach, based only on bedside diagnostic criteria, has been proposed by Kolodny.

Suggested Readings

Kolodny EH: Storage diseases of the reticuloendothelial system. In Hematology of Infancy and Childhood, Chap. 33, Nathan and Oski (edits.). Philadelphia, W.B. Saunders, 1980.
Kolodny EH, Cable WJL: Inborn errors of metabolism. Ann Neurol 11:221, 1982.
McKusick VA: Heritable Disorders of Connective Tissue, 4th ed. St. Louis, C.V. Mosby, 1972.
Menkes JH: Textbook of Child Neurology, 2nd ed. Philadelphia, Lea and Febiger, 1980.
Rosenberg LE, Scriver CR: Disorders of amino acid metabolism. In Metabolic Control and Disease, 8th ed., Chap. 11, Bondy and Rosenberg (edits.). Philadelphia, W.B. Saunders, 1980.
Stanbury JB, Wyngaarden JB, Frederickson DS: The Metabolic Basis of Inherited Disease, 4th ed. New York, McGraw-Hill, 1978.

Chapter 11

The Hyperactive Child and Learning Disorders

Learning difficulties in childhood that appear to be on a neurologic basis do not represent a homogeneous group, nor is there a generally acceptable nomenclature. Various systems to codify these disparate disorders have all met with mixed success; nonetheless, it has been estimated that as much as 5% of the school-age population in the United States fits into this category.

Attempts have been made over the past 5 years to use an intellectual construct similar to that employed in adult behavioral neurology - i.e., localizationist-associationist models of cognitive function. Until such time as these syndromes are better understood, it is perhaps most prudent for the physician to rule out certain treatable medical conditions that may impact or mimic learning disorders, and having done this refer the child for more definitive, usually multidisciplinary, evaluation.

Evaluation

The physician should first try to ascertain which aspects of school performance are most difficult for the child. Is the area of concern pervasive (e.g., the child's ability to concentrate and attend to any task), or are the areas of concern limited to one domain of academic endeavor (such as learning to read)? Armed with some initial concept, a history may then be taken, paying particular attention to the developmental precursors of the issue in question.

A. History

1. Were there prenatal or perinatal factors that might influence the CNS (prematurity, postmaturity, small for dates, intrauterine infection, birth trauma, low APGAR scores)?

2. Is there a family history of individuals with learning disorders, or individuals with surprising job placements? Is there a family history of biologic conditions associated with learning difficulties (non-dextrality, premature greying of the hair, autoimmune disorders)?

3. Is there a provocative developmental history, with motor or language milestones late to appear? Were there oromotor difficulties early in life (excessive drooling, difficulty learning to suck through a straw)?

4. Is there any suggestion of underlying seizure activity (staring spells)?

5. Is there a history of motor overactivity (standardized scales such as the Conners' may help to establish this)?

6. Is there any suggestion of psychological or social turmoil in the family (this may have a significant impact on school performance, but in our experience is usually a diagnosis of exclusion)?

B. Examination

Many examinations that "extend" the range of the traditional neurologic examination have been suggested, and preference for one of these is as much a matter of local option and circumstance as anything. The physician would be best advised to obtain a standard neurologic examination, and then add screening tests for certain domains.

1. The Denver Developmental Screening Test is useful, and quite interobserver reliable; it is suited for children below the age of 6.

2. Hearing should always be screened, particularly if a language disorder is suspected. Seventy-five percent of the children referred to the Learning Disabilities

Clinic at the Children's Hospital (Boston) have not had adequate hearing evaluations prior to being evaluated there.

3. Language screening in children older than age 6 may be readily performed by the administration of the Rapid Automatized Naming, NCCEA Word Fluency, and Boston Naming Tests. These examinations take relatively little time (roughly 10 minutes in a less-than-cooperative 6-year-old, less in older and more cooperative children), are standardized for age and sex, and can be readily learned by the physician. They can allow for rapid triage to a speech-language pathologist if results are significantly aberrant.

4. Unless one has more formal training, standardized intelligence testing is best left to trained psychologists.

5. The assessment of impulsivity and activity is better made on the basis of history, as many hyperactive children perform quite well in a structured office setting. The Conners' scale, or informal parent and teacher observations, are generally more useful.

6. Rarely, more serious neurologic disorders may present as learning problems. Thought should be given to testing for amino acidopathies, thyroid dysfunction, lead, muscular dystrophy, or degenerative diseases if the history or exam suggests these.

C. Treatment

Treatment is usually best left in the hands of individuals familiar with the classroom setting. In the presence of associated language or other specific learning difficulties, we have not found that medications such as Ritalin (methylphenidate) have been particularly successful. That is, we have found them of benefit only in children with "pure" attentional disorders. In those instances, significant behavior modification programs are so often of benefit, that we find only roughly one-third of these patients require medication. Alternative stimulants (Cylert, Dexadrine) or low-dose tricyclic agents may also be tried.

Chapter 12

Coma

Evaluation of the comatose child depends upon physical examination and history obtained from family and friends. One attempts to find a treatable cause of coma. Treatable causes include ingestions, metabolic derangements, and at times supratentorial processes, e.g., acute epidural or subdural hematoma. Anatomically, coma implies bilateral hemisphere dysfunction (e.g., drugs, metabolic factors, meningitis), temporal lobe herniation and compression of brainstem (e.g., intracerebral tumor), or brainstem dysfunction (e.g., compression from a posterior fossa mass). If certain basic points are established when examining the comatose child, the extent of structural central nervous system (CNS) derangement and sometimes the cause can be determined.

Observe the Child Carefully

1. Is there decorticate posturing (arms flexed at elbows), implying bilateral hemisphere dysfunction but an intact brainstem?

2. Is there bilateral decerebrate posturing (extension of legs and arms), implying bilateral damage to structures at the upper brainstem or deep hemisphere level?

3. Is the child yawning, swallowing, or licking his lips? Does he appear comfortable as if sleeping? If so, coma cannot be very deep and major brainstem function is probably intact.

4. Are there repetitive, multifocal myoclonic jerks?
   These are characteristic of anoxic or metabolic
   encephalopathy.

5. Are there multifocal seizures? These are often seen in
   infections and metabolic encephalopathies.

WHAT IS THE RESPIRATORY PATTERN?

Cheyne-Stokes respiration implies bilateral
hemisphere dysfunction with an intact brainstem and may be
the first sign of transtentorial herniation; it also
accompanies metabolic disorders and congestive heart
failure. For reasons poorly understood, it is seldom seen
in childhood.

Central neurogenic hyperventilation (rapid deep
breathing) usually indicates damage to the brainstem
tegmentum between midbrain and pons.

Apneustic breathing consists of a prolonged
inspiratory cramp followed by an expiratory pause and is
usually seen in pontine damage.

Ataxic (irregular) breathing is a terminal event
signifying disruption of medullary centers.

Remember, extensive damage to the brainstem is
rarely accompanied by a normal breathing pattern.

Coma with hyperventilation frequently signifies a
metabolic derangement:

. Metabolic acidosis: diabetes, uremia, lactic
  acidosis, poisoning.

. Respiratory alkalosis: salicylates, hepatic failure.

. Combined metabolic acidosis, respiratory alkalosis -
  Reye's syndrome.

DOES THE CHILD RESPOND TO EXTERNAL STIMULI?

1. Apply a truly noxious stimulus to determine whether the
   child is unresponsive. Noxious stimuli may cause
   decorticate or decerebrate posturing and thus give a
   clue to the level of brain damage. Are there
   asymmetries?

2. Check for a response of the limbs to pain. Is there a low level reflex such as flexion, extension, or adduction? Is there asymmetry? Abduction of shoulder or hip is usually not reflex and indicates that higher level (cortical) function is present.

3. Test for a voluntary response -- e.g., let the child's hand fall toward his face and see if he resists.

EXAMINE THE PUPILS CAREFULLY?

1. A metabolic (not structural) cause is usually present if a comatose child has no response to external stimuli, absent doll's eyes, and corneal reflexes, but preserved pupillary responses. In many cases, he has ingested a barbiturate.

2. Glutethimide (Doriden) ingestion and atropine poisoning result in large unreactive pupils that may be indistinguishable from a structural lesion.

3. Reactive pupils imply an intact midbrain. Midbrain damage produces pupils 5 to 6 mm in size that do not react to light but may fluctuate in size (hippus).

4. Pontine damage produces pinpoint pupils that react to bright light when viewed with a magnifying glass. Heroin and pilocarpine also produce pinpoint pupils.

5. A unilaterally fixed, dilated pupil is seen with damage to the third nerve, often after it has left the brainstem.

//Third nerve palsy may mean
transtentorial herniation.//

This is a valuable sign of temporal lobe (uncal) herniation from a supratentorial lesion (see Chap. 22).

CHECK FOR CORNEAL REFLEXES AND DOLL'S EYES

Absence of corneal reflexes and doll's eyes means pontine damage or, in the case of ingestion, dysfunction. If there is no doll's eye response, use ice water irrigation with the head elevated 30 degrees (be sure there is no wax in the ears or a perforated tympanic membrane); tonically deviated eyes to the side of the irrigation, a normal response, signifies that certain parts of the brainstem are functioning (see Fig. 25.2).

Do not check for doll's eyes response in trauma patients until cervical spine films have been obtained.

MOTOR SYSTEM EXAMINATION

Hyperreflexia and upgoing toes are seen in meningitis, hypoglycemia, Reye's encephalopathy, and structural lesions (e.g., subdural hematoma); downgoing toes are often seen with drug ingestions or other metabolic causes. Hemiplegia suggests a structural CNS lesion.

LABORATORY STUDIES

Laboratory studies must be carried out to exclude metabolic causes of coma such as hyper- or hypoglycemia, drug ingestion, hypercalcemia, uremia, Reye's syndrome, and electrolyte disturbance. Ferric chloride may be used to screen the urine for possible ingestion. It is purple in the presence of aspirin and ketones, green with phenothiazines, isoniazide, and high concentrations of epinephrine. When clinically appropriate (e.g., signs of meningeal irritation), lumbar puncture is indicated to rule out infection or bleeding in the CNS; intoxications, Reye's syndrome, or bacterial abscess are relative contraindications to lumbar puncture.

//Hypoglycemia is one of the most treatable causes of coma.//

Remember: hypoglycemia is one of the most treatable causes of coma. After drawing a blood glucose, give all children with coma of unknown etiology 50% glucose intravenously when first seen.

Treatment must include:

1. Guarantee airway: via intubation, if necessary.

2. Maintain blood pressure.

3. Proper positioning to avoid aspiration.

IRREVERSIBLE COMA

It is frequently necessary to establish whether irreversible coma has occurred. This state ws originally defined according to the "Harvard criteria" (JAMA 205;337, 1968) as follows: (1) total unawareness or unresponsiveness to externally applied stimuli; (2) total absence of spontaneous movement or respiration; (3) no reflexes, no brainstem function; and (4) a flat EEG. These criteria have undergone a number of revisions. A diagnosis of irreversible coma or cerebral death should not be made by house officers. Appropriate neurologic consultation and great caution are required. When poisoning, metabolic dysfunction, or hypothermia may be involved, such criteria may be invalid. Cerebral flow studies may also be useful.

Suggested Readings

Guidelines for the determination of death. JAMA 246:2184, 1981.

Mofenson HC, Greensher J: The unknown poison. Pediatrics 54:336, 1974.

Plum F, Posner J: Diagnosis of Stupor and Coma, 3rd ed. Philadelphia, F.A. Davis, 1979.

Prensky AL: Neurologic metabolic emergencies in infants and young children. In Critical Care of Neurologic and Neurosurgical Emergencies, Thompson RA and Green JR (edits.). New York, Raven Press, 1980.

Scherz RG: The differential diagnosis of coma due to poisoning and exogenous toxins. Paediatrician 6:190, 1977.

Chapter 13

Headache

A careful history is crucial in evaluating the child with headache. Although great reliance is placed on the parental descriptions, it is equally important to have the <u>child</u> describe his headache. Most children over the age of 5, and some younger, can give a coherent description of their headache and associated symptoms.

In evaluating the child with headache the pediatrician must rule out organic causes:

1. On neurologic examination check for focal signs that might suggest a structural lesion. Be sure to visualize the fundi.

2. Listen for bruits. Although bruits are common in childhood and usually of no significance, bruits that are asymmetrical or continuous may result from an underlying arteriovenous malformation.

3. If the child develops a stiff neck during a severe headache, suspect subarachnoid hemorrhage and perform a CAT scan, and if negative, an LP. Meningitis (viral, bacterial, fungal, or tuberculous) often presents with headache and stiff neck.

• Remember, headache and stiff neck (especially head tilt) may be seen with tumors or other processes in the posterior fossa. Always check fundi before performing an LP, and if there is a question of papilledema, obtain a CAT scan prior to LP.

5. Headache is one of the first signs of meningeal leukemia.

6. In a child with cyanotic heart disease who develops prominent headache, suspect a brain abscess.

7. Hydrocephalus may cause headache (check head circumference).

8. Check for hypertension – this may be associated with headache.

9. Examine ears and teeth carefully.

10. Pseudotumor is a cause of headache.

Apart from organic causes, the basic differential in the child with headache is between vascular or migraine headaches and functional or tension headaches (see Table 13.1). Migraine may occur in children as young as 2 years of age. Functional headaches do not occur until the latter part of the 1st decade.

Migraine is a common complaint (approximately 5% of children). In the child under 5 it may present as episodes of pallor and vomiting unassociated with a recognizable illness; the episode is usually followed by sleep and rapid recovery. When the child is able to talk, he may describe an associated headache. Many children quickly learn the best treatment, i.e., sleep.

In the older child, careful questioning may elicit a history of a visual aura where none was volunteered, i.e., bright spots, bright lines, flashes, blurring, "pieces missing"; the child may draw a scotoma better than he can describe it.

Migraine may either be classic (preceded by visual or other prodrome) or common (no prodrome). The latter has the same character as classic migraine but develops with no warning and builds up slowly. Both are associated with scalp tenderness and photophobia.

//Migraine headaches are "sick" headaches.//

Nausea and vomiting are also prominent in migraine -- thus, the designation "sick headaches." The gastrointestinal disturbance usually occurs after the headache has been established.

Table 13.1

Migraine/vascular	Functional/tension
Throbbing	Non-throbbing, often vividly described
Bifrontal, hemicranial, occipital	Frequently vertex or poorly localized. May be diffuse, "everywhere."
Occasional visual aura, i.e., scintillating scotoma, spots, and bright lights.	No warning
Occurs in paroxysms or attacks. Trouble-free intervals.	Constant, daily, for long periods.
Associated symptoms: nausea and vomiting, photophobia, vertigo	Depression, light-headedness, "dizziness" but not true vertigo.
Neurologic complications: transient hemiplegias, aphasias, sensory symptoms, ophthalmoplegia.	Neurologically normal
Positive family history for vascular headaches or car sickness.	Not common
May wake child from sleep.	May be associated with insomnia
Positive response to appropriate medication.	Medication usually ineffective

Classic migraine begins with a visual prodrome such as flashing lights, blind spots, or hemianopsia. Headache begins when the visual prodrome is over, usually in 20 minutes. In complicated migraine other symptoms occur -- e.g., difficulty talking, tingling of face or extremities, or actual hemiparesis ("hemiplegic migraine"). Occasionally ophthalmoplegia is seen during the course of complicated migraine (ophthalmoplegic migraine").

Common migraine or classic migraine with only a visual aura requires no workup beyond a careful history and physical examination. Complicated migraine (hemiplegia, aphasia, oculomotor palsy) requires a more extensive investigation to rule out an organic lesion. Be suspicious if migrainous attacks are always one-sided; migraine that has occurred on both sides is almost always benign.

Confusional episodes may occur in juvenile migraine and actually be the presenting complaint; confusional migraine is a diagnosis of exclusion and requires a basic workup (EEG, LP, CAT scan, and screen for toxic or metabolic encephalopathies, including Reye's syndrome).

Migraine is believed to have a vascular-biochemical basis and to have two phases; vasoconstriction, sometimes associated with an aura, followed by vasodilation and headache. There may be an associated electrical disturbance, especially in the prodromal period. Thus, EEGs are frequently abnormal in migrainous children and the EEG interpretation in isolation might suggest a seizure disorder or structural abnormality. There is a small but definite association between migraine and seizures and both may occur in an individual or family. The combination of seizures plus migrainous or other headache syndromes warrants further investigation (e.g., CAT scan).

TREATMENT

1. It is important to discuss the diagnosis of migraine with both child and parents, since it is a recurrent problem.

2. Preadolescents with frequent, incapacitating migraine are best treated with prophylactic phenobarbital (15

to 30 mg twice daily) and an analgesic, e.g., aspirin, at the onset of the headache. An analgesic alone is sufficient if the headaches are not severe.

3. In young children, if phenobarbital does not help, diphenylhydantoin (100 to 150 mg/day) or ergonovine maleate (0.25 mg each morning) may be tried. Cyproheptadine (Periactin), 2 to 4 mg given 2 to 3 times/day depending on age, may also be of benefit. Methysergide (Sansert) has not been used regularly in children and is not recommended because of its side effects. Amitriptyline or other tricyclic agents may be of benefit if administered in small doses (10-30 mg every night).

4. In teenagers, Cafergot may be effective if there is a recognizable aura and it can be given before the headache is established. A single dose is taken at the first sign of the aura and repeated 30 minutes later. If ineffective, further doses are of no help. Younger children are generally not helped by Cafergot. Ergonovine maleate (0.25 mg) given as a single dose in the morning for brief periods may be effective. Sublingual preparations, suppositories, or inhalants can be of value when nausea and vomiting are prominent.

5. Propranolol (Inderal) has gained wide acceptance as a migraine prophylactic in adults and children with incapacitating, recurrent headaches (contraindicated in children with asthma or cardiac disease). Dosage is 60 mg/day under 35 kg, and up to 120 mg/day over 35 kg. Propranolol does not help acute headache.

6. In the older child and teenager, combinations of a rapid acting barbiturate for sleep induction with aspirin-phenacetin-codeine (e.g., Fiorinal) may be of benefit for the actual headache. It is not useful unless the patient is willing to try to sleep. Beware of abuse potential and give limited prescriptions.

7. Amitriptyline in low doses (10-75 mg every night) is quite effective.

8. For difficult to control migraine in the teenager, methysergide (Sansert) may be given prophylactically. It is given for only 3 months at a time because it may cause retroperitoneal fibrosis.

9. Per rectum medication to help induce sleep is helpful when nausea complicates oral treatment, e.g., Nembutal or phenergan suppositories.

10. Prostaglandin inhibitors have recently been shown to be effective. Phenytoin (Dilantin) and carbamazepine (Tegretol) are effective in children with associated seizures or abnormal EEGs.

11. Biofeedback has proven very useful in children with intractable migraines and avoids the dangers of drug habituation.

Precipitating factors include menses, missed meals, excitement, or postexcitement let down, oral contraceptives in teenagers, alcohol, disordered sleep habits, and at times certain foods (chocolate, cheese, or nuts, nitrates, monosodium glutamate).

Headaches associated with depression are difficult to treat with standard "headache medication." Treatment generally requires mild analgesia and an attempt to deal with the stressful life situation that is associated with the headaches. Sometimes antidepressants (amitriptyline, Elavil) and psychotherapy are needed. Amitriptyline has been reported to be of benefit for migraine in adults, even where depression is not a factor, perhaps due to its serotonin actions.

The approach to children with intractable, nonperiodic (everyday, all day) headaches is difficult. An approach to a similar psychosomatic symptom (abdominal pain) is given by Stickler (Am J Dis Child 133:486, 1979), and this approach is equally useful for children with headache.

Suggested Readings

Barlow CF: Headaches and Migraines in Children. Spastics International Medical Publications, Oxford, Blackwell, 1984.
Basser KS: The relation of migraine and epilepsy. Brain 92:285, 1969.
Ling W, Oftedol G, Weinberg W: Depressive illness in childhood presenting as severe headache. Am J Dis Child 120:122, 1970.

Chapter 14

Spinal Cord

The features of spinal cord dysfunction are: (1) a sensory level, (2) a level of motor weakness, (3) no facial (i.e., cranial nerve) involvement, (4) urinary malfunction. Breathing difficulties may be seen, depending on level of injury. Spinal cord dysfunction may be congenital (Table 14.1) or acquired.

TABLE 14.1

CONGENITAL SPINAL CORD ABNORMALITIES

1. Spina bifida occulta: bony abnormalities only. Usually involves the posterior arch of L5-S1 and is asymptomatic. There often is an overlying abnormality of the skin (tuft of hair, dermal sinus, discoloration, or nevus).

2. Spinal dysraphism: more extensive bony abnormalities plus underlying spinal cord malformation; often with an overlying skin abnormality as with spina bifida occulta.

3. Meningocele: meninges protrude to the surface through a bony defect.

4. Myelomeningocele: spinal cord and meninges protrude to the surface through a bony defect. The spinal cord is dysplastic (myelodysplasia).

124

CONGENITAL

The signs of cord involvement will depend on the level of the lesion, e.g., thoracic lesions will be associated with upper motor neuron signs in the legs - spasticity, increased deep tendon reflexes, and upgoing toes. Lumbar cord abnormalities usually show lower motor neuron signs - weakness, absent deep tendon reflexes, atrophy, orthopaedic deformities such as club foot, and prominent urinary difficulties.

Myelomeningocele usually affects the lower spine and signs in the lower extremities include hypotonia, areflexia, decreased sensation, distended bladder, and patulous anus. Hydrocephalus is frequently associated.
In diastematomyelia, a congenital septum (occasionally calcified) bisects the cord in an anterior-posterior direction. The bony spicule may be seen on plain films of the spine. Surgery may prevent progression of symptoms.

Intraspinal lipomas and other tumors may be associated with lumbar bony abnormalities. In a child with spinal cord dysfunction, plain films of the spine are mandatory. Ultimately a myelogram may be needed for definitive diagnosis. MRI of the spine is frequently quite successful for localizing lesions.

ACQUIRED

Spinal cord transection may occur in difficult deliveries, especially breech; the cord is stretched and damaged, usually in the lower cervical area. These babies are often in respiratory distress, and their clinical picture may be mistaken for the respiratory distress syndrome. Total lack of tone in the lower extremities with active use of the upper extremities is diagnostic of cord transection. Sensory and sweat levels can be demonstrated; unusual hand posturing is often present. Myelography may be necessary for diagnosis. Treatment is conservative.

SPINAL CORD COMPRESSION

Acute spinal cord compression is a neurologic emergency.

Characteristic Symptoms

- Back pain.

- Paresthesias in legs ("funny feeling," tingling, or numbness).

- Change in urinary function (child urinates more or less frequently, dribbles, priapism).

- Weakness in lower extremities (especially climbing stairs).

- Constipation.

Early Signs

- Loss of pinprick sensation or a different reaction to pinprick in the lower extremities. The child may or may not have a sensory "level" to pinprick.

- Loss of position or vibration sense in the feet.

- Slight hyperreflexia in the lower extremities as compared to the upper (Note: the toes may be downgoing and reflexes reduced in early acute cord compression.)

- Tenderness over the spine is one of the most helpful signs in determining the level of the lesion.

- A sweat level (decreased sweating below the level of the lesion).

Late Signs

- Definite weakness.

- Definite hyperreflexia.

- Upgoing toes.

- A sensory level to pinprick and/or vibration. It is often helpful to check vibration sense up and down the spine in search of a level.

- Loss of anal sphincter tone, absent abdominal reflexes.

CAUSES OF SPINAL CORD COMPRESSION

Epidural Compression

.   Metastases (especially neuroblastoma, leukemia, and lymphoma).

.   Epidural abscess.

.   Epidural hematoma (hemophilia and trauma).

.   Bony abnormalities (achondroplasia); in Morquio's syndrome and trisomy 21 compression occurs at C1-C2.

Extraarachnoid, Intradural Compression

.   Neurofibroma.

Intraarachnoid

.   Seeding from a cerebral tumor (medulloblastoma, ependymoma, or ectopic pinealoma).

.   Dermoid cyst.

Intramedullary Compression

.   Glioma.

.   Ependymoma.

.   Hemato- or hydromyelia.

DIAGNOSTIC STEPS

1.   Perform a careful neurologic examination; estimate the level of the cord lesion.

2.   Check for primary tumor sites, e.g., careful abdominal examination, chest x-ray, and complete blood count (CBC). Perform body scan (CAT) and ultrasound when indicated.

3.   Early consultation with a neurologist and/or neurosurgeon is necessary.

4.   Remember that if an LP is performed and viscous fluid is obtained (due to the high protein associated with

cord compression), the needle should <u>not</u> be removed; use it to inject contrast material for the myelogram.

5. Do not proceed with the LP if pus is encountered; this may signify epidural abscess and organisms must not be introduced into the subarachnoid space.

TREATMENT

Treatment depends on the site(s) of cord block and the etiology. Radiotherapy (for lymphoma), surgical decompression (for extradural tumors), or a combination of both is used.

Give intravenous dexamethasone (0.25 mg/kg up to 10 mg) immediately (before myelograpy, radiotherapy, or surgery) when compression is suspected as it may help preserve spinal cord function.

NOTE

1. <u>Discitis</u>, an inflammatory condition of the nucleus pulposus, may mimic a spinal cord tumor and present with back, hip, leg, or abdominal pain, refusal to walk, meningeal irritation, and rigidity of the spine. It is usually seen in children under age 5, although it may occur until teenage years. It is associated with an elevated sedimentation rate, eventual narrowing of the disc space, and, occasionally, calcification of the disc space. Spine compression by striking the heel or head may cause pain at the involved site. L4-L5 is most frequently involved. Discitis is generally benign and responds to rest and antibiotics.

2. The syndrome of <u>acquired scoliosis</u> in childhood and adolescence is usually idiopathic, especially in girls, and may be familial. Films of the spinal column are otherwise normal and there are no associated neurologic signs.

//Abnormal neurologic signs or scoliosis in a boy should lead to careful investigation and consideration of myelography.//

Check carefully for dermatologic manifestations of neurofibromatosis (cafe-au-lait spots).

3. <u>Transverse myelitis</u> is characterized by the acute or subacute development of paraplegia, occasionally

asymmetrical, associated with back pain and sensory loss. It may or may not be related to a preceding exanthem (e.g., chickenpox) or viral illness (e.g., mononucleosis). The cerebrospinal fluid may show pleocytosis with increased protein and normal sugar. Myelography is often necessary to rule out a compressive lesion. Treatment is conservative. Corticosteroids are often used when the etiology is thought to be postinfectious and/or demyelinating.

4. The long term management of children who are paraplegic requires a multidisciplinary approach with particular attention to the bladder and bowel, active physical therapy, and careful orthopaedic follow-up.

Suggested Readings

Altrocchi PH: Acute transverse myelopathy. _Arch Neurol_ 9:111, 1963.

Bresnan MJ, Abroms IF: Neonatal spinal cord transection secondary to intrauterine hyperextension of the neck in breech presentation. _J Pediatr_ 84:734, 1974.

Crichton JH: Acute spinal cord disease in childhood. _Dev Med Child Neurol_ 23:643-646, 1981.

Editorial: Mechanisms in scoliosis. _Lancet_ 2:1234, 1976.

Matson DD: _Neurosurgery of Infancy and Childhood_. Springfield, IL, Charles C Thomas, 1969.

Rocco HD, Eyring EJ: Intervertebral disc infections in children. _Am J Dis Child_ 123:448, 1972.

Chapter 15

Hyperreflexia and Hyporeflexia

Pathologically hyperactive reflexes imply disease between cortex and anterior horn cells in the spinal cord, and hypoactive reflexes imply disease between spinal cord anterior horn cells and muscle.

HYPERREFLEXIA

Some children have exaggerated relexes that might be considered hyperactive. Symmetrically hyperactive reflexes in the presence of downgoing toes are usually normal. If hyperactive reflexes truly reflect pyramidal tract disease, the toes should also be abnormal. The presence or absence of a Babinski response in children can be difficult to interpret because of withdrawal. Thus, the Chaddock maneuver (stroking the dorsolateral aspect of the foot) may be used to elicit a Babinski response. Also, contraction of the tensor fascia lata when the sole of the foot is stroked suggests pyramidal tract dysfunction rather than withdrawal. Abdominal reflexes (stroke skin next to umbilicus) may be absent on the side of pyramidal tract dysfunction. Check for the presence of a jaw jerk in children with hyperreflexia; its presence suggests bilateral lesions above the midpons affecting the motor division of the fifth cranial nerve.

A unilaterally upgoing toe or one-sided hyperreflexia implies damage to one side of the nervous system. Decide whether this represents an old lesion or a new one.

Check for:

1. <u>History</u> <u>of</u> <u>Difficult</u> <u>Birth</u> <u>or</u> <u>Neonatal</u> <u>Complications</u>:
    an otherwise normal child may have unilateral
    hyperreflexia with no apparent cause due to birth
    injury and mild cerebral palsy (see Chap. 4). Look for
    asymmetry in limb size (thumbnail bed asymmetries or
    differing shoe sizes); was there early handedness? If
    the child is left-handed, are there other left-handers
    in the family, or might the left-handedness represent
    early damage to the left hemisphere?

2. <u>Old</u> <u>Neurologic</u> <u>Disease</u>: a child with prior
    meningitis, head trauma (even "uncomplicated"),
    subdural hematoma, etc., may have unilateral
    hyperreflexia.

3. If the history suggests <u>newly</u> <u>developing</u> <u>signs</u> <u>or</u>
    <u>symptoms</u>, a full investigation is warranted.

    Hyperreflexia in arms and legs implies a lesion at the
    cervical cord or higher; <u>hyperreflexia</u> <u>in</u> <u>legs</u> <u>only</u>
    implies a lesion below the cervical cord. There are
    three exceptions to this anatomic rule:

1. <u>Cerebral</u> <u>Palsy</u>: leg fibers may be selectively
    involved in the white matter of the hemispheres,
    giving increased reflexes in legs only ("spastic
    diparesis"). This is typically seen in premature
    infants (perinatal-telencephalic leukoencephalopathy).
    Alternatively, hypotension may affect the parasagittal
    border zone area (between middle and anterior cerebral
    arteries) affecting grey and white matter. This is
    more typically seen in full terms.

2. <u>Hydrocephalus</u>: hydrocephalus may present as spastic
    diparesis because parasagittal leg fibers are
    stretched most by dilated ventricles.

3. <u>Parasagittal</u> <u>Intracranial</u> <u>Mass</u>: by virtue of its
    location, it affects cortical leg fibers, producing
    hyperreflexia in legs only, and mimics a cord lesion.
    Headache, personality change, and seizures may be
    present. Tumors in this location are uncommon in
    childhood, but those involving the corpus callosum may
    do so as can the more common deep midline tumors
    (craniopharyngioma, pinealoma, dysgerminoma) by
    bilateral pressure or hydrocephalus.

NOTE: Diffuse hyperreflexia can be seen in metabolic and toxic encephalopathies, e.g., early Reye's syndrome, uremic, hepatic, and lead encephalopathy.

Bilateral Hyperreflexia

This implies bilateral pyramidal tract dysfunction. In children, possibilities include:

1. Spinal Cord Compression: look for primary spinal cord tumor (check x-rays for interpedicular distance, erosions), bony abnormalities (diastematomyelia, congenital scoliosis of the spine), or secondary involvement by non-CNS tumors (dumbbell intraforaminal tumor or neuroblastoma). Morquio's syndrome, achondroplasia, and trisomy 21 can also be associated with spinal cord compression. Check for sensory level, local back tenderness, skin abnormalities (hemangiomas, tuft of hair, peau d'orange) (see Chap. 14).

2. Familial Spastic Paraplegia: check for other affected family members.

HYPOREFLEXIA

Hyporeflexia usually indicates peripheral nerve disease, although it is seen if any component of the reflex pathway is abnormal: peripheral nerve, sensory root, anterior horn cells in cord, motor root, or muscle. Reflexes can be reinforced by having a child pull his hands apart, make a fist, or bite down. Areflexia implies no reflexes, even with reinforcement; reflexes present only with reinforcement imply an intact reflex pathway and may or may not be abnormal. Consider the following points when confronted with hyporeflexia:

Normally Hypoactive Reflexes: occasionally one sees otherwise normal children with hyporeflexia and no obvious cause. The biceps jerk is often difficult to obtain in young children. In premature infants especially, but also in full term infants, triceps jerk reflexes are normally difficult to demonstrate.

Spinal Shock: areflexia may be seen during the initial acute stages of cord damage -- whether traumatic, vascular, or neoplastic. Hyperreflexia then usually supervenes.

Acute Hemiplegia: initially there may be hyporeflexia on the side of the hemiparesis; later hyperreflexia.

Asymptomatic Areflexia with Large Pupils: this is a benign syndrome (Adie's), consisting of areflexia and large pupils that react to accommodation but not to light.

Riley-Day Syndrome: these children have areflexia, hypotonia, relative indifference to pain, increased sweating, absent tears, drooling, and recurrent pneumonias.

Myopathy: in later stages, muscle disorders may be associated with hyporeflexia (although usually not areflexia until late in the course). Remember, weakness from muscle disease is generally proximal (shoulder and hip), while weakness from peripheral nerve disease is usually distal (hand and foot).

For the same degree of weakness a motor neuropathy can be differentiated from a myopathy by the absence of reflexes.

Isolated Unilaterally Absent Reflex: this is most often seen with diseases affecting specific peripheral nerves or roots (see Chap. 17).

Bilateral Areflexias Associated with Neuropathies: this broad category of diseases affects peripheral nerves and causes areflexia. If one cannot elicit reflexes, the child usually has a neuropathy.

Bilateral Areflexia Associated with Spinal Muscular Atrophy: the variants of Werdnig-Hoffmann disease will present with areflexia, fasciculations of the tongue, and normal intelligence. The autosomal recessive disorder is usually rapidly fatal

ACUTE INFECTIOUS POLYNEURITIS (GUILLAIN-BARRE SYNDROME)

Areflexia with subacutely developing ascending motor weakness and minimal sensory loss is the classic presentation of the Guillain-Barre syndrome. There may be tingling or "funny feelings" in hands and feet. Check for a history of a recent infection or surgery, since infectious polyneuritis may begin 7 to 14 days after a systemic infection (usually viral, often infectious mononucleosis) or may follow surgery.

Clinical Characteristics: in the mild form, motor difficulties are confined to gait difficulties and trouble using upper extremities. The moderate form is merely an extension of the mild form but includes enough weakness that the child is now unable to walk alone. In the severe form, the ascending paralysis involves respiratory muscles and cranial nerves. These children may require intubation, tracheostomy, and intensive respiratory care. Improvement begins within 2 weeks in 60% of cases and within 3 weeks in 85%. They do not progress further, and the clue to the diagnosis is areflexia. Most children recover completely and walk again. Certain autonomic phenomena are seen acutely with Guillain-Barre syndrome including hypertension and cardiac arrhythmias. The Miller Fisher variant (areflexia, external ophthalmoplegia) may be seen in children.

Diagnosis: look for ascending muscle weakness that is more prominent proximally, areflexia, a mild distal sensory loss and bilateral facial weakness (an important clue). An LP usually shows the diagnostic raised CSF protein without pleocytosis. (CSF protein may be normal during the first week, warranting a retap). Nerve conduction velocities are usually delayed, although they may be normal early in the course.

Treatment: in Guillain-Barre syndrome, the ultimate severity of the paralysis may not be evident at first. Therefore, carefully monitor respiratory function until the paralysis has reached a plateau. How high can the child count on one breath? Check vital capacity and blood gases.

//Monitor respiratory function
when Guillain-Barre is suspected.//

Steroids are of questionable benefit: a brief trial may be indicated if the child's condition is rapidly deteriorating. Plasmapheresis is being evaluated as a possible treatment modality, but given the relatively benign nature of the childhood form, plasmapheresis may be of limited utility.

Workup: check for toxin exposure, tic paralysis, diphtheria (palatal and extraocular muscle palsies, myocarditis), botulism (blurred vision), myasthenia gravis, polymyositis, and polyarteritis; these processes may mimic the Guillain-Barre syndrome. Also, test for mononucleosis, hepatitis, and mycoplasmal infection; they may represent the preceding illness.

CHARCOT-MARIE-TOOTH DISEASE (PERONEAL MUSCULAR ATROPHY)

Charcot-Marie-Tooth disease is the prototypical familial neuropathy. These children have minimal early sensory loss, a widespread areflexia not confined to the legs, pes cavus, and ultimately, distal atrophy ("champagne-bottle" legs). Inheritance is autosomal dominant. Family histories may not be positive because cases with minimal involvement occur. Always examine the parents for areflexia and cavus feet. Familial neuropathies blend into other inherited neurologic diseases, with other signs present, e.g., neuropathy plus cerebellar dysfunction, nystagmus, and ataxia (Friedreich's ataxia); neuropathy plus tremor (Roussy-Levy syndrome).

WORKUP OF NEUROPATHIES

In most instances the etiology of a child's neuropathy is clear. Check the following points when dealing with a neuropathic process of undetermined cause:

1. Is there evidence of toxin exposure: arsenic (painful red feet and gastrointestinal disturbances), thallium (alopecia), lead or other metals (copper, zinc, and mercury)? Consider organic toxins (phosphates and solvents). Tic paralysis?

2. Check for drugs that may cause neuropathy. Nitrofurantoin, isoniazid, and vincristine are common offenders.

3. Does the child have an associated systemic illness: infectious mononucleosis, lupus erythematosus, or polyarteritis?

4. Is the neuropathy relapsing? This form of polyneuritis often responds dramatically to steroids.

5. Perform nerve conduction studies when the diagnosis is in doubt; nerve conduction velocity is decreased in most peripheral neuropathies and is most markedly decreased in demyelinating neuropathies (polyneuritis, Charcot-Marie-Tooth disease) and less so in axonal neuropathies (Friedreich's ataxia).

Suggested Readings

Dubowitz V: Muscle Disorders in Childhood. Vol. 16 of Major Problems in Clinical Pedriatics. Philadelphia, W.B. Saunders, 1978.

Dyck PJ, Thomas PK, Lambert EH: Peripheral Neuropathy. Philadelphia, W.B. Saunders, 1975.

Evans OB: Polyneuropathy in childhood. Pediatrics 64:96, 1979.

Guillain-Barre syndrome. Ann Neurol 9(Suppl): 1981.

Kuban KCK, et al: Deep tendon reflexes in premature infants. Pediatr Neurol 2:266-271, 1986.

Chapter 16

Myopathy

When confronted with a child who may have a myopathy, the pediatrician must establish whether the weakness is indeed myopathic, if the myopathy is congenital or acquired, and if acquired, whether it represents a manifestation of another illness, e.g., thyroid disease.

HISTORY

In a child with weakness in whom the diagnosis of myopathy is made, one finds:

1. The weakness is usually gradual rather than sudden in onset.

2. Climbing stairs and running are particularly difficult (proximal weakness).

3. There is an absence of paresthesias or "pins and needles" feeling in the limbs.

4. Bowel and bladder function are not affected.

Establish the following points:

1. Is there a <u>family history</u> of a similar disorder? (If possible, examine parents and siblings; unsuspected cases may be found.)

2. Is there myotonia of grip (i.e., inability to relax after a firm contraction)?

3. Is there trouble swallowing (often seen in
    polymyositis) or variation in weakness during the day
    (myasthenia)?

PHYSICAL EXAMINATION

The child with a myopathy often presents with these
findings:

1. Proximal limb strength is more impaired than distal
    strength (except in myotonic dystrophy). Check
    deltoids (shoulder) and iliopsoas (hips). Weakness
    tends to be distal in neuropathies. CSF protein is
    normal in myopathies.

2. Gower's Sign: child "climbs up" his legs with his
    arms when going from lying to standing because of hip
    and gluteal weakness.

3. Neck flexion is weaker than neck extension.

4. Reflexes are preserved or slightly decreased except in
    late stages of the disease.

5. Sensation is unimpaired in contrast to neuropathies.

6. Wasting may be present, although there are no
    fasciculations.

Check these points, which help distinguish one
myopathy from another:

1. Note whether facial muscles are involved. Have child
    shut eyes tight, puff cheeks, or attempt to whistle
    (difficult in facioscapulohumeral dystrophy).

2. Check for fatigability (myasthenia), especially if
    eyes are involved (ptosis and extraocular palsies).

3. See if pelvic and thigh muscles are more involved than
    those of the head and shoulders (limb-girdle
    dystrophy).

4. Check for myotonia by percussing the thenar eminence
    or the tongue and check for lid myotonia by having the
    child shut his eyes tightly and then quickly try to
    open them. Lid lag may be present. Children with
    myotonia are often unable to "let go" after a
    handshake.

5. Hypertrophy may be part of certain dystrophies, e.g., Duchenne's (80%), limb-girdle (20%).

LABORATORY STUDIES

Characteristic features of myopathies include:

.   Elevated creatine phosphokinase (CPK) levels (aldolase, serum glutamie oxaloacetic transaminase (SGOT), and lactic dehydrogenase (LDH) may be elevated, check isozymes).

.   Normal CSF, including protein.

.   Electromyogram (EMG) shows myopathic changes.

.   Normal nerve conduction velocity.

.   Abnormal muscle biopsy. It is important to pick a moderately affected muscle and ensure proper collection and study of the biopsy material.

MUSCULAR DYSTROPHY

The term dystrophy implies a progressive course with destruction and loss of muscle, although not all muscular dystrophies are associated with a dire prognosis. Accurate diagnosis is important for day-to-day management, prognosis, and genetic counseling.

A. Pseudohypertrophic Muscular Dystrophy (Duchenne's Dystrophy)

This is the prototype dystrophy. Onset is early in the 1st decade, most children are nonambulatory by early in the 2nd decade (ages 10 to 13), and death usually occurs by age 20. Most children never learn to run or walk normally. Inheritance is sex-linked recessive although many new cases are thought to be sporadic, i.e., secondary to a high mutation rate. Nonetheless, complete family screening, including CPK levels of the mother and her sisters, may indicate more widespread carrier states. The familial incidence has been reduced by genetic counseling and because affected males do not survive to reproductive age. Genetic mapping: Recent studies have localized the gene for Duchenne's.

//Screen slow walkers (18 months) for dystrophy.//

Affected children have very high CPK levels (10 to 100 times normal) that precede clinical signs. This provides a valuable method for early screening of male siblings. Similarly, carrier females will frequently have elevated CPK levels (1 1/2 to 2 or more times normal). A rare female carrier will show mild clinical signs (Lyon hypothesis). Carrier detection is best accomplished in childhood. Thus, check the sisters of affected boys early. Diagnosis is made on the basis of hypertrophy of calf muscles, marked elevation of CPK, family history, and clinical course. The EKG is often abnormal from the onset, showing large right precordial R waves and deep Q waves in left precordial leads.

Treatment is directed toward maintaining mobility (physical therapy, night casts, and braces). Tendon lengthening procedures are occasionally indicated. The latter must not be accompanied by prolonged bed rest and convalescence, as inactivity or immobilization seems to increase disability. Terminal complications relate to infection (pneumonia) and/or cardiac failure.

B. Benign Sex-Linked Recessive Dystrophy (Becker Type)

A group of children has been identified in whom symptoms are phenotypically similar to Duchenne's dystrophy, but the disease is milder. The onset is later, and children remain ambulatory until adult life. There are pseudohypertrophic changes and moderately elevated CPK levels (not as high as in Duchenne's dystrophy). Such males can reproduce; thus an affected boy may have an affected grandfather.

C. Facioscapulohumeral Dystrophy

Facioscapulohumeral dystrophy (FSH) begins late in the 1st or early in the 2nd decade, progresses very slowly, and may cause only minimal disability. Facial and scapular weakness may be asymmetrical, and triceps and/or biceps may be weaker than deltoid muscles. Inheritance is autosomal dominant. Families may not view FSH as a disability, and the discovery of unsuspected cases in relatives is common. FSH rarely can present as a Mobius syndrome (bifacial weakness) in infancy and have a malignant (severe) course with early disability. There may be an associated sensory-neural hearing loss.

Table 16.1 (Part 1)
MUSCULAR DYSTROPHIES

	Inheritance	Age of onset	Course	Enzyme (CPK)
Duchenne	Sex-linked recessive (many sporadic cases)	3-6	Rapid, inability to walk within 10 yr, death by age 20	Marked elevation
Becker (benign sex-linked recessive)	Sex-linked recessive	4-30	Benign, variable disability	Mild to moderate elevation
Facioscapulohumeral (Landouzy-Dejerine)	Autosomal dominant	7-12	Benign, abortive cases common. Minor disability	Normal
Limb-girdle (Erb's)	Autosomal recessive, occasionally dominant	5-10	Intermediate, disability in 30's and 40's	Usually normal
Central core	Autosomal dominant (sporadic)	Infancy	Usually nonprogressive, delayed motor milestones, later mild to moderate weakness	Normal
Nemaline (Nema is the Greek word for thread)	Autosomal dominant with variable penetrance	Variable, infancy to childhood	Non- or slowly progressive (occasionally fatal cases in infancy)	Normal
Myotubular	Autosomal recessive	Infancy	Slowly progressive	Usually normal
Myotonic dystrophy (Steinert)	Autosomal dominant	Variable (infancy to 50's)	Variable, depending on age of onset	Normal
Myotonia congenita (Thomsen)	Autosomal dominant	Infancy	Benign	Normal

Table 16.1 (Part 2)
MUSCULAR DTSTROPHIES

Unusual features	Cardiac	Histology	Electron microscope
Pseudohypertrophy, lower IQ's, toes may be upgoing	R and Q wave changes	Severe dystrophic changes with cellular infiltration	No unusual features
None	? None	Dystrophic changes often less marked, ringbenden	No unusual features
Inability to pucker lips	None	Mild myopathic changes	No unusual features
Face occasionally involved, occasional hypertrophy, deltoids often spared	Rare	Myopathic changes	No unusual features
Hypotonia (floppy baby)	None	Central cores devoid of enzyme activity (Type I fibres)	Decreased mitochondria in core
Marked hypotonia, elongated face, high arched palate, arachnodactyly	None	Nemaline bodies in continuity with Z-band	Abnormal Z-band material
Facial diplegia, ptosis and ocular palsies	None	Myotubes, central nuclei	Myelin figures and mitochondria in tubule
Myotonia, baldness, cataracts, mental retardation, impotence, distal weakness	Conduction abnormalities	Myopathic, sarcoplasmic inclusions, ringbenden, central nuclei	No unusual features
Myotonia which decreases with use. Strong and well muscled	None	Large fibers affected	No unusual features

D.   Limb-Girdle Dystrophy (Erb's Dystrophy)

This term (and eponym) refers to a diverse group of muscle disorders; many are included only because they clearly do not fit elsewhere. It is from this group that most recent subgroups have been identified. Inheritance is autosomal recessive. Onset is late in the 1st and 2nd decades. Mild cases with later onset also occur. Occasional confusion arises with Duchenne's dystrophy because of associated hypertrophy (20% of cases of limb-girdle dystrophy), and this may also explain suspected sporadic cases of Duchenne's dystrophy in females. CPK levels are usually not as elevated as in Duchenne's dystrophy; muscle biopsy is characteristic.

E.   Congenital Myopathies

A group of myopathies manifests in infancy as a "floppy infant." Children have delayed motor milestones and nonprogressive weakness. These myopathies have been defined by unique histologic and histochemical features: (1) central core - a central area of the muscle fiber with reduced enzyme activity; (2) nemaline - abnormal Z-band material in the shape of rods; (3) myotubular - central nuclei. See Table 16.1 for an outline of their clinical features.

NOTE: Arthrogryposis multiplex congenita, congenital fixation, or ankylosis of one or more joints is associated with fetal immobility usually secondary to either myopathic or neural dysfunction in utero. Such children should be worked up accordingly, i.e., enzymes, electromyogram, nerve conduction velocities, and muscle biopsy.

F.   Kugelberg-Welander Disease (Late Onset Juvenile Spinal Muscular Atrophy)

This disorder begins in the 1st or 2nd decade and can mimic a myopathy because it presents as proximal weakness and wasting. Unlike a myopathy, however, reflexes are markedly diminished or absent and CPK levels are only minimally elevated. It is now known to be a disease of anterior horn cells and probably represents a continuum of Werdnig-Hoffmann disease (infantile spinal muscular atrophy), which occurs at an older age and with a slower progression. Muscle biopsy and electromyogram show neurogenic rather than myopathic features. Autosomal recessive inheritance is assumed.

CONDITIONS ASSOCIATED WITH MYOTONIA

Myotonia is the inability to relax a muscle after a contraction. It is demonstrated most easily when the child attempts to relax his hand after a grip or to relax facial muscles that have contracted (after looking up, lid lag may be seen). It can also be demonstrated by percussion of either the tongue or the thenar eminence. The electromyogram demonstrates a characteristic "dive-bomber" sound, an electrical phenomenon, that may be present in the absence of clinical myotonia.

A. Myotonia Congenita (Thomsen's Disease)

This rare condition is usually inherited as an autosomal dominant trait. Myotonia is generalized and is not accompanied by weakness. In fact, affected children usually have striking muscle hypertrophy (infant Hercules) and good strength, especially after a few contractions.

B. Myotonic Dystrophy (Steinert's Syndrome)

Myotonic dystrophy is a systemic disorder. The fully developed clinical picture includes cataracts, frontal balding, testicular atrophy, diabetes mellitus, and heart disease; as such it is usually seen in adults. Myotonic dystrophy is unique because weakness is more prominent distally. Children usually present as hypotonic (floppy) infants (see Chap. 3) with facial diplegia and feeding difficulty or weakness. They often have delayed eye opening after crying. There may be mental retardation. Inheritance is autosomal dominant.

C. Periodic Paralyses; Paramyotonia Congenita (Eulenburg's Disease)

Most children described as having "paramyotonia," i.e., myotonia on exposure to cold or episodic attacks of weakness, suffer from one of the periodic paralyses.

1. Hypokalemic Periodic Paralysis: symptoms begin late in the 1st or during the 2nd decade. Attacks of paralysis begin after rest (often after sleep) with weakness beginning in the legs and then ascending; deep tendon reflexes may be absent during an attack. Exercise, large meals, or exposure to cold may precipitate attacks and improvement begins a few hours after the attack. EMG shows electrical silence.

Serum potassium falls to very low levels during a major attack. Strength and potassium levels are normal between attacks, although repeated attacks may cause residual weakness. Inheritance is autosomal dominant.

2. <u>Hyperkalemic Periodic Paralysis</u>: occurs at an earlier age than the hypokalemic form, and clinical characteristics are similar (attacks after rest or sleep). Meals, however, do not provoke weakness, but may even help shorten or prevent attacks. Myotonia, especially lid lag, may be present between attacks. Inheritance is autosomal dominant. (A normokalemic form has been reported in patients with a craving for salt, which can be provoked by potassium administration.)

If periodic paralysis is suspected, testing to produce hyperkalemia or hypokalemia is performed. Spironolactone is helpful in the treatment of the hypokalemic form, and acetazolamide (Diamox) is useful in both the hypo- and hyperkalemic forms. <u>Note</u>: Periodic paralysis is associated with hyperthyroidism; thus, thyroid studies should be done. Secondary periodic paralysis may be seen in children with potassium depletion or accumulation, e.g., chronic diarrhea or renal failure. Rarely, a constant cardiac arrhythmia may be associated with periodic paralysis; such cases have a high mortality rate.

MYASTHENIA GRAVIS

Myasthenia gravis is a rare condition in childhood. Its pathophysiology relates to a postsynaptic defect of acetylcholine receptors at the neuromuscular junction most probably caused by circulating antibodies. Three forms are recognized:

1. Transient neonatal myasthenia gravis affects approximately 10% of infants of mothers with myasthenia and usually clears within 3 weeks after birth coincident with the clearing of placentally transferred antibodies (there is a reported 10% mortality). Manifestations include feeding difficulty, weakness, and, less commonly, ptosis. Management consists of <u>respiratory support</u> and cautious use of anticholinesterase medication for the duration of symptoms. In severe cases, exchange transfusion may be of benefit. Do not overtreat.

2. Permanent congenital myasthenia gravis is rare and not associated with maternal myasthenia. The presenting symptoms are the same as those in transient myasthenia. Prolonged therapy is necessary but may be of minimal benefit. It is not associated with receptor antibodies but has been demonstrated to be a structural abnormality at the neuromuscular junction; six subtypes have been posited.

3. Childhood myasthenia (onset after 1 year) resembles myasthenia in adults, can be severe, and includes ptosis, ophthalmoplegia, generalized weakness, dysphagia, and occasionally respiratory difficulties. Circumscribed cases occur in which only the eyes are affected. Girls significantly outnumber boys in all series.

   If the diagnosis is suspected, an intravenous edrophonium (Tensilon) test (0.2 mg/kg, maximum 10 mg) is indicated. Because of uncomfortable side effects (lacrimation, sialorrhea, and abdominal cramps) that may induce crying, intramuscular neostigmine (Prostigmin) (0.04 mg/kg) is often used in children. Atropine will reverse these side effects and should be available (0.01 mg/kg/dose; 0.4 mg maximum). Occasionally, it is necessary to use oral medication in a clinical trial.

1. Remissions are unusual in children with onset under the age of 1 year, but are common with onset after age 1.

2. Oral medications commonly used are neostigmine and a longer acting preparation, pyridostigmine (Mestinon). Restricted cases (ophthalmoplegic) may not require treatment.

3. ACTH and steroids are now standard treatment in disabled adolescents and adults, but their efficacy in childhood is not yet established.

4. Thymectomy is of benefit for children who do not respond to medication and who are significantly disabled.

DERMATOMYOSITIS/POLYMYOSITIS

   Polymyositis is an inflammation of muscle associated with the insidious onset of proximal muscle weakness, elevated muscle enzymes and sedimentation rate, and inflammatory changes on biopsy. Treatment is with steroids.

In addition to polymyositis, the features of dermatomyositis are: an erythematous butterfly rash of the face, a heliotrope rash of the eyelids, and scaliness of the extremities, especially over the knuckles. Histologically, there is a prominent arteritis. Dermatomyositis is associated with systemic involvement, especially of the gastrointestinal (GI) tract (dysphagia, abdominal pain, and upper and lower GI bleeding); diffuse subcutaneous calcium deposits are common. Treatment with steroids and antimetabolites may be effective. The prognosis is variable.

Polymyositis and dermatomyositis in children are not associated with malignancy as in adults. Isolated polymyositis in children less than 10 years of age is unusual.

TREATMENT OF MYOPATHIES AND ASSOCIATED DISORDERS

Only supportive treatment is available for children with muscular dystrophy; diagnosis is crucial for genetic counseling. Treatable causes of secondary myopathic weakness include:

1. Endocrine: hyper- and hypothyroidism and Cushing's disease.

2. Myopathy associated with systemic lupus erythematosus or rheumatoid arthritis.

3. Periodic paralyses.

4. Myasthenia gravis.

5. Drug induced: especially steroid myopathy.

6. Infection: trichinosis and toxoplasmosis.

Suggested Readings

Bohan A, Peter JB: Polymyositis and dermatomyositis. N Engl J Med 292:344, 403, 1975.

Donaldson JO, et al: Antiacetylcholine receptor antibody in neonatal myasthenia gravis. Am J Dis Child 135:209, 222, 1981.

Dubowitz V: Muscle Disorders in Childhood. Vol 16 of Major Problems in Clinical Pediatrics. Philadelphia, W.B. Saunders, 1978.

Pachman LM, et al: Juvenile dermatomyositis. J
Pediatr 96:226, 1980.

Walton JN: Disorders of Voluntary Muscle, 4th ed.
London, Churchill Livingstone, 1981.

Chapter 17

Peripheral Nerve and Root Dysfunction

To diagnose peripheral nerve and root injuries, one must determine which muscles are affected and the nature of the sensory loss. Thus, one must know which roots and nerves supply which muscles and the sensory distribution.

ROOTS AND MUSCLES (Table 17.1)

There is an overlap between roots and the muscles they supply; thus, more than one root generally innervates each muscle. Nevertheless, certain muscles serve as standard clinical indices for each root so that if one particular root is out, there should be one muscle (or muscle group) that is particularly weak.

Each root has a sensory distribution as represented on the standard dermatome chart (see Fig. 25.9).

REFLEXES (Table 17.2)

Reflexes are diminished in root and peripheral nerve disease. There are four primary reflexes to remember, with particular roots and muscles necessary for their function. An easy way to learn the roots is to remember that, going from ankle to triceps, the roots are numbered consecutively from one to eight (Table 17.2).

Table 17.1
ROOTS AND THE PRIMARY MUSCLES THEY SUPPLY

Root	Muscle	Action
C5	Deltoid	Shoulder abduction
C5	Infraspinatus	Humeral external rotation
C5,C6	Biceps	Supinated forearm flexion
C6	Extensor carpi radialis and ulnaris	Wrist extension
C7	Extensor digitorum Triceps	Finger extension; forearm extension at elbow
C8,T1	Interossei and lumbricales	Digital abduction and adduction (check: have child move fingers apart and together against resistance)
L2,L3,L4	Quadriceps Iliopsoas Adductor group	Knee extension Thigh on hip flexion Thigh adduction
L5	Anterior tibial and extensor hallucis	Ankle and large toe dorsiflexion (check: have child walk on heels)
S1	Gastrocnemius	Ankle plantar flexion (check: have child walk on tiptoes)

Table 17.2
THE FOUR PRIMARY REFLEXES

Reflex	Roots needed for reflex	Muscle carrying out the reflex
Ankle jerk	S1	Gastrocnemius
Knee jerk	L2, L3, L4	Quadriceps
Biceps	C5, C6	Biceps
Triceps	C7, C8	Triceps

Table 17.3
CHARACTERISTIC FEATURES
ASSOCIATED WITH VARIOUS NERVES

Nerve	Involvement
Median	Thumb and thenar eminence
Ulnar	Little finger and hypothenar eminence
Radial	Wrist drop
Femoral	Absent knee jerk (weak hip flexion and knee extension)
Peroneal	Foot drop
Sciatic	Pain down lateral thigh, often absent ankle jerk

NERVES AND MUSCLES OF THE UPPER EXTREMITY (Table 17.3)

Median Nerve

The median nerve (C6-T1) originates in the shoulder (brachial plexus) and supplies two basic muscle groups:

1. Forearm: pronator of the forearm, radial flexion, and wrist abduction.

2. Hand: thumb flexion, abduction, and opposition; index and middle finger flexion; and first two lumbricales (proximal joint flexion and distal joint extension).

    Sensory loss involves the thumb and first two fingers.

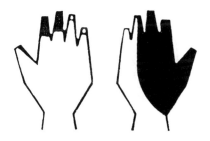

Clinical Comment: a complete median nerve lesion (both forearm and hand muscles) is usually secondary to traumatic injury in the axilla. Partial involvement may be seen with damage at the wrist.

When median nerve involvement is suspected, think of thumb and thenar eminence.

Ulnar Nerve

The ulnar nerve (C8-T1) is the counterpart of the median nerve in the forearm and hand. It supplies all muscles and sensory areas (on palm) not supplied by the median nerve. When ulnar nerve disease is suspected, think of little finger and hypothenar eminence.

> //Ulnar nerve = little finger
> Median nerve = thumb//

The ulnar nerve wraps around the medial aspect of the elbow and supplies the following two muscle groups:

1. Forearm: ulnar flexion at the wrist.

2. Hand: ring and little finger flexion: little finger abduction and opposition, all the interosseous muscles (used to spread fingers apart and bring together), third and fourth lumbricales, thumb adduction.

Sensory loss involves the fourth and little finger.

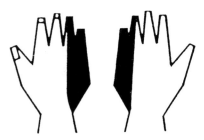

Clinical Comment: ulnar nerve palsy gives a "claw hand" deformity affecting the ring and little fingers. The ulnar nerve is most commonly injured at the elbow where it is superficial. A claw hand is also seen with involvement of C8-T1 roots at the origin of the brachial plexus, e.g., due to trauma or surgery. Check for Horner's syndrome (small pupil and ptosis) on the same

side as the claw hand. This indicates sympathetic system
involvemnt near the roots of the brachial plexus (T1).

Radial Nerve

The radial nerve (C5-C8) winds around the lateral
aspect of the elbow. When one suspects radial nerve
involvement, think of wrist drop.
The radial nerve supplies these muscles:

1. Supinator of the forearm.

2. Extensors of the fingers, wrist, elbow (triceps), and
   thumb.

Sensory loss involves the back of the hand and is not
always present.

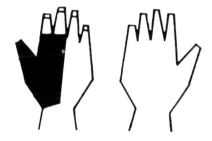

Clinical Comment: injury to the radial nerve may
occur in the axilla (e.g., after using crutches or by a
fractured humerus) resulting in inability to extend the
elbow plus wrist drop. If the radial nerve is involved at
the elbow, only wrist drop is found. In radial nerve
palsy, ability to spread fingers apart (ulnar nerve
function) may be weak due to the mechanical disadvantage
caused by the wrist drop. Check with wrist resting on a
flat surface (e.g., table) to overcome that handicap.

Brachial plexus injuries may occur during difficult labor.

1. Erb: upper brachial plexus, fifth and sixth cervical root affecting shoulder and biceps. The diaphragm (C3, 4, 5) may occasionally be involved. Good prognosis.

2. Klumpke: lower brachial plexus, C8-T1, affecting forearm flexion and small muscles of the hand. A Horner's syndrome may be present. Myelography may reveal avulsion of roots. Poorer prognosis. Be sure to rule out associated fractures (clavicle or humerus).

Note: Bilateral brachial plexus injuries are almost invariably associated with spinal cord damage.

NERVES AND MUSCLES OF THE LOWER EXTREMITY (Table 17.3)

Obturator Nerve

The obturator nerve (L2-L3-L4 roots, ventral portion) supplies the adductors of the thigh.

Femoral Nerve

The femoral nerve (L2-L3-L4 roots, dorsal portion) supplies the iliopsoas (hip flexion) and quadriceps (knee extension). Dysfunction usually results in a diminished or absent knee jerk. Femoral nerve involvement may be distinguished from root involvement at L2-L3-L4 (e.g., by paravertebral tumor) by checking thigh adduction (obturator), which is affected if L2-L3-L4 roots are involved but spared if the femoral nerve alone is involved. Causes of femoral neuropathy include injury during attempted femoral artery puncture, pelvic trauma, and pelvic surgery. There may be bleeding into the lumbosacral plexus in hemophilia.

Lateral Femoral Cutaneous Nerve

This pure sensory nerve (L2-L3) supplies the lateral thigh. There is tingling, burning, and pain. The lateral femoral cutaneous nerve syndrome (meralgia paraesthetica) is rare in children but is seen in adolescents, especially related to pressure from casts, or tight trousers.

Sciatic Nerve

The sciatic nerve (L4-S3) supplies hamstring (flexion of knee) and all muscles below the knee.
At the knee it divides into the:

1. Peroneal nerve, which runs anteriorly around the head of the fibula and supplies muscles that dorsiflex and externally rotate the foot, and sensation on top of the foot.

2. Tibial (posterior) nerve, which runs posteriorly at the knee, supplies muscles of plantar flexion and internal rotation of the foot, and sensation on the sole of the foot.

Injection Injuries: the sciatic nerve may be injured during attempted intramuscular injection in the buttock. The initial palsy may be relatively complete, but recovery is usual and often the main residual weakness involves only the lateral portion of the sciatic nerve (the portion closest to the site of injection in the upper quadrant), causing a foot drop.

Irritation of any root from L4-S3 may produce sciatica, a sensory disturbance beginning in the buttock and radiating down the lateral aspect of the thigh. The most common cause of sciatica is lumbar disc protrusion, often with reflex loss, pain, and weakness in a root distribution (see Table 17.4). Lumbar disc protrusions occur in adolescence and almost invariably have a history of antecedent trauma: scoliosis may be a feature. Straight leg raising, coughing, and sneezing often aggravate the pain. In some adolescents there may be no abnormal neurologic findings with a herniated disc.

The decision to carry out myelography and/or surgery for lumbar discs depends on the inability to relieve pain with bed rest and the presence of weakness or other abnormal neurologic signs. Root tumors (neurofibromata) can mimic a disc syndrome. Loss of sphincteric control constitutes an emergency.

Peroneal Nerve

The peroneal nerve supplies dorsiflexors (tibialis anterior) and everters (turning out) of foot. Inverters (turning in of the foot) are not supplied by the peroneal nerve but by the posterior tibial nerve. The sensory distribution involves the lateral aspect of the leg and dorsum of the foot.

Clinically, peroneal nerve palsy results in foot drop and is analogous to wrist drop (radial nerve) in the upper extremity. It is a frequent pressure palsy (due to the superficial location of the nerve at the lateral aspect of the knee) -- either from trauma or pressure in a thin or comatose child. Hereditary peroneal neuropathy (Charcot-Marie-Tooth disease) is associated with bilateral foot drop, a wasted anterior leg compartment below the knee, and pes cavus. Remember, peroneal palsy spares the inverters of the foot; if they too are weak, the lesion is higher, generally at the roots, sciatic nerve, or cord.

Posterior Tibial Nerve

This nerve is rarely injured alone as it runs deep in the calf.

INVESTIGATION OF NERVE AND ROOT DYSFUNCTION

Examine the child to determine whether the nerve or root is involved. Determine whether the sensory loss (or symptom) and muscle weakness (if present) fit the distribution of a particular nerve or root.

Establish the etiology. If a particular nerve or root is definitely involved, determine the specific etiologic factors unique to that nerve or root.

Important to ask:

1. Did a nerve palsy come on after sleep or surgery (pressure palsies, injections)?

2. Is there evidence of trauma, old or new?

3. What are the child's activities and habits that might predispose to a particular neuropathy?

4. Is there evidence of systemic disease, e.g., allergic neuropathy affecting the brachial plexus (brachial neuritis), polyarteritis, eremia, Epstein-Barr virus or diphtheritic infection, or treatment with a neuropathic agent such as vincristine?

SEVENTH NERVE PALSIES, INCLUDING BELL'S PALSY

Peripheral involvement of the seventh cranial nerve is a well recognized syndrome in childhood and adolescence.

Table 17.4

MOST COMMON LUMBAR DISC SYNDROMES

Root	Root exits at interspace*	Reflex affected	Motor weakness	Sensory changes (if any)	Straight leg raising
L4	L4-L5	Knee jerk	Knee extension	Anterior thigh	−
L5	L5-S1	Posterior tibial may be helpful	Large toe dorsi-flexion	Large toe	+
S1	S1-S2	Ankle jerk	Foot, plantar flexion	Foot, lateral border	+

* A nerve root is usually compressed by a lateral disc at the interspace of root exit or by a more medial disc at the next higher interspace.

Onset is often heralded by facial pain; diagnosis is based on demonstrating complete facial nerve involvement, i.e., paralysis of both lower face and forehead, in the absence of other neurologic findings. Central lesions that affect fibers prior to their synapse in the seventh nerve nucleus in the brainstem spare forehead musculature. In addition to innervating facial musculature, fibers from the seventh nerve innervate the lacrimal gland of the eye, the stapedius muscle in the ear (hyperacusis), the submaxillary and sublingual glands, and carry afferent taste fibers from the anterior two-thirds of the tongue. The majority of cases are idiopathic (Bell's palsy). The most common recognizable cause is an associated otitis or mastoiditis. Other causes include infectious mononucleosis, the Guillain-Barre syndrome (bilateral seventh nerve palsies, see p. 156), pontine glioma (other cranial nerve nuclei are involved, especially the sixth, see p. 161), skull fracture, severe hypertension, diabetes, sarcoid and histiocytosis, and post-exanthema or following immunization. Seventh nerve palsy in infants may be seen after a difficult delivery or as a part of the Mobius syndrome (a congenital anomaly affecting seventh and sixth nerve nuclei in the brainstem). Melkersson's syndrome is recurrent seventh nerve palsies associated with facial edema.

Treatment with prednisone often significantly reduces the amount of residual facial disfiguration in the idiopathic variety and should be given within the first 72 hours of onset: over age 10, 40 mg for 4 days, taper off over the next 4 days; under age 10 begin with 20 mg. Patching the eye and methylcellulose eye drops will help prevent corneal ulceration. Surgical decompression is of no benefit except in mastoiditis. Recovery usually begins within 1 to 4 weeks of onset and may take longer than 3 months to be complete. Children with hyperacusis and loss of tearing have a poorer prognosis; taste loss does not appear to affect prognosis.

Suggested Readings

Adour KK: The bell tolls for decompression. N Engl J Med 292:748, 1975.

Aids to the Examination of the Peripheral Nervous System Injuries. London, Her Majesty's Stationery Office, 1976.

Sunderland S: Nerves and Nerve Injuries, 3rd ed. London, Churchill Livingstone, 1979.

Wolf SM, et al.: Treatment of Bell palsy with prednisone: prospective, randomized study. Neurology 28:158, 1978.

Chapter 18

Malignancy and the Nervous System

Primary intracranial tumors in childhood are predominantly infratentorial, i.e., located in the posterior fossa (cerebellum, brainstem). Metastatic intracranial disease is rare in childhood; when present it is usually due to leukemia or lymphoma.

Signs and Symptoms of Posterior Fossa Tumors

1. Headache is often prominent. Young children usually do not complain of headache, and persistent headache in young children should be regarded with suspicion.

2. Ataxia and gait difficulties are common because the cerebellum or cerebellar tracts are usually involved. In addition, hydrocephalus secondary to obstruction by tumor affects leg fibers that are in close proximity to the dilated frontal horns. Ataxia may be truncal or involve the extremities. There may be hypotonia and decreased reflexes with cerebellar involvement or lower limb hyperreflexia with brainstem involvment and/or hydrocephalus.

3. Vomiting occurs secondary to raised intracranial pressure or direct effects on medullary centers. In infants, irritability may be the primary symptom of raised intracranial pressure.

4. Papilledema occurs secondary to increased intracranial pressure and may be acute or chronic. It is mandatory to examine the fundi of children suspected of tumor or raised intracranial pressure; this may require

restraining and sedating the child and/or dilation of the pupils. Be certain to used short acting mydriatics and note on the chart that they have been used.

5. Hydrocephalus is common in posterior fossa tumors because of the obstructed cerebrospinal fluid (CSF) flow. Head circumference may be increased, and when the head is percussed, there may be a characteristic "cracked pot" sound. Skull films may show separated sutures (up to age 13) or localized erosion of bone, especially in the sellar regions.

6. Diplopia due to a sixth nerve palsy may be present. The palsy is usually caused by raised intracranial pressure and is of no localizing value.

7. Stiff neck, head tilt, or torticollis may be associated with involvement of infratentorial structures.

    //Ataxia and head tilt are signs of posterior fossa tumor until proven otherwise.//

8. Personality changes may be the first sign of an intracranial neoplasm, especially with pontine gliomas. Children may have received a psychiatric evaluation prior to the appearance of the first cranial nerve palsy.

9. Pyramidal tract signs and cranial nerve palsies are the hallmarks of brainstem tumor. Note: unless there is hydrocephalus, upgoing toes are generally seen late in the course of cerebellar tumors.

SUPRATENTORIAL TUMOR

    Seizures and hemiparesis are distinguishing features of supratentorial tumors, two features generally absent in infratentorial malignancies. Occasionally a supratentorial tumor will present with ataxia, presumably due to involvement of fronto-ponto-cerebellar fibers. Supratentorial tumors also cause raised intracranial pressure (vomiting, headache, and papilledema).

SPECIFIC TUMOR TYPES IN THE POSTERIOR FOSSA

A. Medulloblastoma: is one of the most malignant infratentorial tumors, arising from the midline portion of the cerebellum. It occurs in the 1st decade, with peak incidence between 3 and 6 years. Treatment includes attempts at surgical excision (at which time tissue diagnosis is made) and radiation of the head and the entire neuraxis (medulloblastoma frequently seeds along the subarachnoid space to the spinal cord). Many children die within 2 years; recent advances in radiotherapy have significantly improved survival rates.

B. Cerebellar Astrocytoma: is the "benign" tumor of the posterior fossa. The age incidence is similar to medulloblastoma. Unlike medulloblastoma, cerebellar astrocytoma is noninvasive and does not seed along the subarachnoid space. Cerebellar astrocytomas are often cystic and can be totally removed at surgery; radiation therapy is generally not necessary.

C. Ependymoma: generally occurs in the fourth ventricle and because of its location is often impossible to remove totally. Vomiting, sometimes before the development of papilledema, is an early presenting feature. Occasionally ependymomas present as subarachnoid hemorrhage. These tumors generally occur in the 1st decade. Radiation therapy is given becaused ependymomas may seed down the neuraxis; long term survival is uncommon.

D. Brainstem Glioma: occurs in the latter part of the 1st decade, in children older than those with cerebellar medulloblastomas or astrocytomas. Clinical features include bilateral cranial nerve palsies, cerebellar dysfunction, and early pyramidal tract signs. There often is a preceding psychiatric history.

> //Multiple cranial nerve palsies, long tract signs, and no raised intracranial pressure = brainstem glioma.//

Obstruction of CSF flow, hydrocephalus, and papilledema usually do not occur until late in the course. Surgical excision is impossible. Diagnosis is made by the characteristic clinical picture, CAT scan (with contrast), or MRI that shows an enlarged brainstem. Despite radiation therapy, most of these children die within 1 to 2 years. Dexamethasone is a useful palliative medication. (Some children with presumed brainstem gliomas have survived after radiation and brainstem size has returned to normal. It is suspected that the process in some of these children was infectious or demyelinating rather than neoplastic.)

OTHER PRIMARY BRAIN TUMORS

A. Glioma of Cerebral Hemisphere: occurs throughout the first 2 decades, and in contrast to posterior fossa tumors, often presents with seizures and/or hemiparesis. There may be raised intracranial pressure, and signs depend on the tumor's location. CAT scan or MRI is needed for diagnosis; treatment and prognosis depend on the location and cell type of the tumor. There is an increased incidence of intracranial gliomas in children with tuberous sclerosis and neurofibromatosis.

B. Craniopharyngioma: is a suprasellar tumor that occurs throughout childhood. Because of its location, presenting signs and symptoms include: (1) features of raised intracranial pressure secondary to obstruction of CSF flow in the area of the third ventricle; (2) pituitary dysfunction, especially growth retardation; and (3) visual field deficits secondary to involvement of the optic tracts. Occasionally the tumor may extend into the cerebral hemispheres or hypothalamic region. Craniopharyngiomas in children invariably are associated with suprasellar calcification - thus, a routine skull film generally suggests the diagnosis. Treatment includes surgery and radiation therapy. Long term survival is the rule.

C. Hypothalamic Glioma is a rare childhood tumor which may cause the "diencephalic syndrome." Children are affected during the first 3 to 4 years of life and present with failure to thrive and marked loss of subcutaneous fat, but they appear bright and alert. Eye signs (nystagmus), disc changes, and occasionally elevated CSF protein distinguish them from other children with failure to thrive. Diagnosis is by CAT scan or MRI; no treatment is available other than radiation.

D. Optic Glioma: presents as impaired visual acuity, strabismus, proptosis or exophthalmos, optic atrophy, or papilledema. Skull films usually show an enlarged optic foramen. Optic gliomas are associated with von Recklinghausen's disease where they are frequently bilateral. Treatment of this slow growing tumor is controversial; some advocate surgery, some radiation, and others feel conservative follow-up is best, especially in neurofibromatosis.

LABORATORY

Diagnosis of intracranial malignancies requires CAT scan or MRI and often surgery. Lumbar puncture (LP) is dangerous in children with posterior fossa tumors or hydrocephalus. Phase reversal on the EEG often suggests supratentorial tumors; it may be normal with infratentorial lesions. Skull films can be diagnostic (craniopharyngioma) or suggest raised intracranial pressure (split sutures, sella changes). CAT scan is the best noninvasive procedure for diagnosis of intracranial lesions.

TUMORS OF THE SPINAL CORD

Primary tumors of the spinal cord are uncommon. Symptoms include leg weakness, back pain, neck spasm, urinary difficulties, and leg numbness. Signs include weakness, hyperactive reflexes with extensor plantars, a sensory level, spine tenderness to percussion, and scoliosis (see Chap. 14). Secondary extrinsic spinal cord involvement, e.g., via neuroblastoma or lymphoma, produces a similar clinical picture. Myelography is the definitive diagnostic procedure. Surgical decompression often prevents paraplegia.

LEUKEMIA AND LYMPHOMA

These malignant processes are associated with nervous system dysfunction, although they usually do not invade the brain and spinal cord (parenchyma) or present as masses.

Leukemia

Leukemia is associated with a triad of neurologic complications.

1. Leukemic infiltration of meninges (of both brain and spinal cord) and nerve roots is common, and symptoms frequently develop during hematologic remission. Meningeal leukemia presents as headache, nausea, and vomiting. There is raised intracranial pressure, and there may be papilledema. Cranial nerve palsies occur and commonly involve the abducens (sixth) and facial

(seventh) nerves; seizures, visual disturbances, and ataxia may also occur. Diagnosis is made by LP; CSF shows a decreased sugar and an elevated protein. The cytocentrifuge is commonly used to identify leukemic cells. Treatment with intrathecal methotrexate and radiotherapy is effective and is given prophylactically when the child enters hematologic remission; this combined therapy may lead to an encephalopathy.

NOTE: There may be infiltration surrounding cord and roots; look for signs and symptoms of cord compression and root dysfunction.

2. Intracranial hemorrhage occurs in leukemia and is related to a low platelet count (subarachnoid bleeding) and/or a leukocyte count greater than 100,000/mm³ (intracerebral bleeding). In the former, once bleeding has occurred, transfusion therapy is of little benefit. In the latter, treatment is aimed at reducing leukostasis and preventing thrombosis.

3. Infection: these children may develop CNS infection with opportunistic organisms, e.g., fungal (Cryptococcus). When CNS symptoms are present, even if only drowsiness and headache, perform an LP to look for meningeal leukemia or infection. In children with low peripheral white counts, there may be CNS infection with few or no cells in the CSF.

NOTE: Herpes zoster is common, at times affecting roots with prior leukemic infiltration. Pain usually precedes the skin eruption.

Lymphoma

Children with lymphoma are subject to the same complications as those with leukemia except for intracerebral hemorrhage.

Spinal cord compression by progressive lymphoma is especially common, as are compressive syndromes in other parts of the nervous system: brachial plexus, recurrent laryngeal nerve (vocal cord paralysis), phrenic nerve, cervical sympathetics (Horner's syndrome), and lumbosacral roots. The treatment of choice is radiation.

NOTE: Intracranial metastases are rare in children -- they may occur in association with neuroblastoma and nephroblastoma (Wilms' tumor).

Suggested Readings

Hyman CB, Bogle JM, et al: Central nervous system involvement by leukemia in children. _Blood_ 25:1, 1965.

Kornblith PL, Walker MD, Cassady JR: Neoplasms of the central nervous system. In _Cancer Principles and Practice of Oncology_, DeVita VT Jr, Hellman S, and Rosenberg Sa (edits). Philadelphia, J.B. Lippincott, 1982.

Matson DD: _Neurosurgery of Infancy and Childhood_. Springfield, IL, Charles C Thomas, 1969.

Nachman JB, Honig FR: Fever and neutropenia in children with neoplastic disease. _Cancer_ 45:407, 1980.

Neiri RL, Burgert EO, Groover RV, et al: Central nervous system complications of leukemia: a review. _Mayo Clin Proc_ 43:70, 1968.

Weiss WD, Walker ME, et al: Neurotoxicity of commonly used antineoplastic agents. _N Engl J Med_ 291:78, 127, 1974.

Chapter 19

Infections: Meningitis, Encephalitis, and Brain Abscess

A lumbar puncture (LP) is mandatory whenever meningitis is suspected. If it is impossible to perform an LP because of bony abnormalities or local infection in the lumbar area, a cisternal tap by a neurologist or neurosurgeon or placement of a needle under fluoroscopy is indicated. If brain abscess is a real possibility, it may be necessary to delay the LP temporarily pending CAT scan. Remember, a posterior fossa tumor can be associated with a stiff neck (always check fundi).

SYMPTOMS OF MENINGITIS

In newborns and infants the clinical features of meningitis are frequently nonspecific, viz., fever, irritability, cyanosis, lethargy, and a high pitched cry, or poor feeding; there usually is not a stiff neck. The anterior fontanelle may be bulging and there may be seizures. Remember, seizures plus fever demand an LP. Neonatal meningitis is more common in premature infants and is associated with prolonged labor in term babies.

In older infants (after age 1 to 2 years) signs of meningeal irritation appear – stiff neck, headache, positive Kernig's sign (with thigh flexed on abdomen, child resists knee extension), and Brudzinski's sign (attempts to flex the neck result in reflex flexion of the knee and hip).

ETIOLOGY OF MENINGITIS

A. <u>Bacterial</u>: the three most common agents responsible in children are <u>Haemophilus influenzae</u>, <u>Neisseria meningitidis</u>, and <u>Diplococcus pneumoniae</u>. <u>H. influenzae</u> is the most common pathogen below age 5; vaccination is now recommended as part of routine childhood immunizations. Meningococcal meningitis is seen in children and young adults. Pneumococcal meningitis is especially common in children with sickle cell disease. Enteric bacteria (e.g., <u>Escherichia coli</u> and group B beta <u>Streptococcus</u>) are the most common causes of neonatal meningitis.

<u>Tuberculous meningitis</u> is always associated with tuberculous infection elsewhere (miliary, renal, or pulmonary). The clinical presentation may be insidious (headache and low grade fever) or more subacute with a well developed meningeal reaction. Tuberculous meningitis often involves the base of the brain; thus, multiple cranial nerve palsies are seen. Skin testing (PPD) and chest x-ray should be done in all children suspected of meningitis (although both may be negative in tuberculous meningitis). The first clue to tuberculous meningitis may be cerebrospinal fluid (CSF) that shows a neutrophilic response that becomes mononuclear, a consistently low sugar, and no bacterial growth on routine media. Measles vaccination may activate tuberculosis.

B. <u>Fungal</u> Meningitis: usually occurs in the immunologically compromised host – the child with leukemia or on immunosuppressive therapy.

The clinical picture is similar to tuberculous meningitis; fungi can often be identified in India ink preparations of the CSF. Cryptococcal antigen may be identified in the CSF or blood. Most common fungi will grow on regular blood agar if the plates are kept long enough.

C. <u>Viral</u> Meningitis: the hallmark of viral or aseptic meningitis is a mononuclear response in the CSF with a normal sugar. Initially there may be a predominance of neutrophils. Symptoms are similar to bacterial meningitis, although milder. Presentation is often seasonal. The isolation of the virus from the CSF itself is usually difficult, although the diagnosis of a specific viral infection may be made by culturing virus from stool or testing acute and convalescent sera. Mononucleosis is diagnosed by standard laboratory tests. The decision to treat what appears to be a viral meningitis (a neutrophilic response in the CSF with a normal sugar) must be made individually. One may treat until cultures return negative or monitor the untreated child with repeated LPs (N Engl J Med 289:571, 1974).

Note: Mumps meningitis may give a marked pleocytosis with a low sugar (check urinary amylase).

D. Recurrent Meningitis: some children may present with a second or third episode of bacterial meningitis. In these instances (and even in the child with a first episode) certain predisposing factors should be kept in mind:

1. Skull fracture may be the avenue for bacterial entry; the time of head trauma may have been distant from the episode of infection. There may be a history of CSF rhinorrhea (check for a high glucose in nasal secretions).

2. Congenital Sinus Tract: check the skin overlying the entire spine for evidence of a tract, discoloration, or an abnormal patch of hair. In some instances the back of the head must be shaved to find the tract. Recurrent bacterial meningitis with grown negative organisms or Staphylococcus suggest a lumbosacral sinus tract. Recurrent infection with H. influenzae or Streptococcus suggests the Mondiri malformation of the cochlea and adjacent structures.

3. Parameningeal Focus: disease of the mastoids or sinuses, or an epidural infection (of either the spinal canal or the cranial vault) may serve as focus.

4. Children with impaired immune responses are subject to recurrent infections.

CEREBROSPINAL FLUID EXAMINATION (see Chap. 21) (Table 19.1)

Remember, CSF glucose varies with blood glucose levels. It is advisable while collecting CSF to allow a sample to drop directly onto a chocolate agar slant; meningococci may not survive otherwise. If the

Table 19.1

CSF IN MENINGITIS

	Bacterial	Viral	Tuberculous, fungal	Malignant
Cells	200-20,000	Usually less than 200	Often less than 200, may be higher	Often less than 200, may be higher
Cell type	Predominantly polys	Predominantly mononuclear	Predominantly mononuclear	Predominantly mononuclear
Glucose	Low	Normal	Low	Low
Protein	Elevated	Slightly elevated or normal	Elevated	Elevated
Organism	Present	Absent	Present	Absent (Malignant cells)

Remember, there have been many cases of children with bacterial meningitis who had but a few cells on initial LP. In addition, children with sickle cell anemia and leukemia may have bacterial meningitis with only a minimal cellular response.

child has already been placed on penicillin prior to the LP, penicillinase should be added to the culture medium. In partially treated meningitis, diagnosis may be made by measuring bacterial antigens in CSF; this test does not require living organisms. Blood cultures should always be obtained.

NEUROLOGIC COMPLICATIONS

1. Seizures occur in almost one-third of children with meningitis and are most common in H. influenzae meningitis. Recurrent, prolonged, focal seizures that are difficult to control may occur and carry a poor prognosis; they may be due to underlying venous thrombosis, a complicating subdural effusion, or arterial thrombosis. Remember, water intoxication is a metabolic complication of meningitis either from excessive hydration or an inappropriate antidiuretic hormone (ADH) secretion and may present as seizures.

    //Seizures secondary to hyponatremia
    may occur in meningitis.//

2. Cerebral edema is frequently seen in meningitis. Despite the presence of increased intracranial pressure, papilledema is unusual, and, if found, focal complications such as abscess or subdural effusion should be considered. In the absence of papilledema, herniation is seldom seen after LP in meningitis (perhaps because the pressure increase is diffuse and not related to a discrete mass). Nevertheless, remove the minimal amount of CSF needed for study. A sixth nerve palsy may occur secondary to raised intracranial pressure and is not of localizing value. Raised pressure generally resolves early in the course of the illness (within 48 hours), and treatment with agents to reduce pressure (see Chap. 22) is generally not needed. Water intoxication may contribute to raised pressure, especially in the first few days; careful monitoring of serum sodium and osmolarity and judicious administration of fluids are needed.

3. Subdural effusions are commonly seen in children with meningitis under the age of 18 months and should be suspected if there is persistent lethargy, fever, or seizures. All infants with meningitis should be monitored for the presence of subdural effusion by measuring head size and performing transillumination; perform subdural taps if symptomatic effusion is

suspected. Many subdural effusions are asymptomatic and do not require subdural taps. Subdural empyema is rare and is associated with parameningeal infection (e.g., sinusitis and mastoiditis), persistent fever, and focal neurologic signs.

4. Focal Neurologic Signs: arteritis develops in meningitis; thrombosis and subsequent infarction may result in a hemiparesis and often a hemianopsia (usually not seen in uncomplicated subdural effusions). Venous thrombosis usually presents with intractable seizures, focal signs, and blood in the CSF. Basilar meningitis may cause cranial nerve palsies (tuberculosis and fungus). Brain abscess is a rare complication.

TABLE 19.2

ANTIBIOTICS USED FOR MENINGITIS

N. meningitidis	Penicillin G
H. influenzae	Ampicillin and chloramphenicol until sensitivities return and then the appropriate drug (ampicillin being preferred); ceftinazone is an acceptable alternative
S. pneumoniae	Penicillin G
E. coli	Ampicillin and gentamicin or ceftriaxone
Unknown etiology below 2 months:	Ampicillin and gentamicin
Unknown etiology* below 8 years:	Chloramphenicol plus either ampicillin or penicillin
Unknown etiology* above 8 years:	Penicillin or ampicillin

*Assuming no recent head trauma or intracranial surgery, no underlying leukemia or immunosuppressive therapy or subacute bacterial endocarditis.

DOSAGES: Penicillin: 200,000 units/kg/day every
                         4 hours; ampicillin: 300 mg/kg/day;
                         over 1 year, 100 mg/kg/day; - follow
                         blood levels or hematologic
                         indices. Do not use intramuscular
                         forms. Ceftriaxone is an acceptable
                         alternative; dosage for meningitis
                         is 100/mg/kg/day divided twice/day.

NOTE: Gentamicin may have to be given intraventricularly.

PROPHYLAXIS   (Intimate of family contacts only):
                         Meningococcus - Rifampin 20 mg/kg/day,
                         single dose x 2 days; H.
                         influenzae - Rifampin 20 mg/kg/day,
                         single dose x 4 days (give only to
                         children under 3 years).

---

5. Late Complications and Sequelae: communicating and
    noncommunicating hydrocephalus occur in a small number
    of cases, most commonly in infants. Serial measurement
    of head circumference is important for early
    diagnosis. Signs of hydrocephalus usually develop
    within 3 months of the meningitis. Deafness occurs in
    2 to 3% of children with meningitis and may mimic
    retardation. Routine audiologic follow-up (audiometry
    or brainstem auditory evoked responses) is therefore
    indicated. Transient vestibular disturbances can occur
    and present as ataxia. Mental retardation and
    seizures are important sequelae of meningitis.

TREATMENT

1. Monitor metabolic parameters, especially the tendency
    for water intoxication (both iatrogenic and
    inappropriate antidiuretic hormone secretion).

2. Give anticonvulsants if seizures occur (see Chap. 6).

3. Subdural taps when indicated.

4. Steroids in some situations.

ENCEPHALITIS

Viral encephalitis usually presents with fever, altered mental status, seizures, or focal signs. The CSF shows a mononuclear pleocytosis (early there may not be any cells), a normal sugar, and mildly elevated protein (which may occur late). The EEG is usually abnormal. Herpes simplex encephalitis in the older child may present with focal neurologic deficits and complex partial seizures; radioisotope brain scan, CAT, or MRI is indicated because early treatment with acyclovir prevents mortality and morbidity. Diagnosis of encephalitis is based on the clinical picture, CSF findings, and acute and convalescent sera. The child is often treated initially for meningitis. Measles is an important cause of viral encephalitis and is prevented by measles vaccination.

ACQUIRED IMMUNODEFICIENCY SYNDROME (AIDS)

Congenital infection with human immunodeficiency virus (HIV) produces a progressive encephalopathy characterized by failure to thrive with extreme apathy, developmental delay and ultimate regression, apathy hypotonia and basal ganglia and white matter calcification on CAT scan. The brain appears generally wasted and atrophic on CAT scan. The disease presents in the infantile period, in the offspring of an infected mother. While older children (particularly hemophiliacs) may acquire HIV through the routes of infection typical of adults, not enough cases have been studied to determine how they differ from adults with AIDS/AIDS-related complex.

BRAIN ABSCESS

Brain abscess in childhood is usually a complication of infection elsewhere in the body (mastoids, sinuses, or lungs) or of cyanotic congenital heart disease. Brain abscess carries a high morbidity and mortality, but may respond well to therapy depending on its location and the stage at which it is discovered.

Signs and Symptoms

Matson divided the clinical features of brain abscesses into three groups:

1. Infection: brain abscess may present with the characteristic features of an acute central nervous

system (CNS) infection (headache, fever, anorexia, leukocytosis, elevated sedimentation rate, and meningismus). Although LP whould be performed in any child suspected of CNS infection, brain abscess is a major exception.

2. Increased Intracranial Pressure: headache, vomiting, irritability, drowsiness, papilledema, and, in the infant, separation of sutures are common features of raised intracranial pressure. As the abscess increases it acts as a mass lesion and evokes surrounding edema; this causes raised pressure.

3. Focal Neurologic Signs and Symptoms: depending on the location of the abscess, focal signs may develop, including hemiparesis and/or seizures.

Remember, the clinical spectrum of brain abscesses is wide. In the child with an encapsulated abscess, headache is prominent. There may be no signs of infection; the child presents with a slowly evolving focal deficit, seizures, or raised intracranial pressure. Other children are very ill and mimic the child with meningitis.

Diagnosis

The first step in diagnosis is to recognize that brain abscesses occur in certain clinical situations.

1. Congenital Heart Disease: children, especially those with right-to-left shunts, are prone to develop a brain abscess. For reasons poorly understood, brain abscess is rare in children under the age of 2. Remember, children with congenital heart disease are also prone to cerebral thrombosis, although this tends to occur below age 2.

2. Otitis Media: direct extension from a chronically infected ear or from infection in the sinuses or mastoid may be the source of a brain abscess. Spread from the ear is usually to the temporal lobe (check for field deficit); spread from the mastoid is usually to the cerebellum; spread from the frontal sinus is to the frontal lobe.

3. Head Trauma: a fractured skull or bone fragments entering the brain predispose to intracranial infection.

4. <u>Pulmonary</u> <u>Infection</u>: hematogenous spread from bacterial disease of lung (cystic fibrosis) or pleura may result in brain abscess (at times multiple). Pulmonary arteriovenous malformations (Osler-Weber-Rendu) may also be associated with brain abscess secondary to right-to-left shunting.

<u>Lumbar</u> <u>puncture</u> <u>is</u> <u>extremely</u> <u>hazardous</u> <u>in</u> <u>children</u> <u>with</u> <u>brain</u> <u>abscesses</u>:

There is significant incidence of <u>subsequent</u> transtentorial herniation and death when an LP is done in a child with brain abscess. One is not likely to consider an early lumbar puncture in a child with symptoms of increased intracranial pressure and papilledema or with a slowly developing hemiparesis and headache. The possibility of meningitis in a child presents the greatest dilemma. If a brain abscess is a real possibility, we recommend emergency CAT scan with contrast prior to lumbar puncture. If CAT scan is unavailable, EEG and radioisotope brain scan should be performed. These tests are invariably positive in supratentorial brain abscesses (often when arteriography is negative). If the clinical situation demands immediate lumbar puncture, use a small needle and remove minimal fluid. If studies suggest a brain abscess, antibiotics and neurosurgical consultation are needed. Cerebellar and brainstem abscesses may not be seen on early scans or EEG, but generally give signs of a mass in the posterior fossa (headache and vomiting, ataxia, papilledema, and cranial nerve signs in addition to long tract signs). The CSF in brain abscesses may be normal or show a mild to moderate pleocytosis with elevated protein.

TREATMENT

Organisms responsible for brain abscess include <u>Staphylococcus</u> <u>aureus</u>, alpha and beta hemolytic <u>Streptococcus</u>, anaerobic <u>Streptococcus</u>, pneumococci, H. <u>influenzae</u>, and <u>Bacterioides.</u> Appropriate antibiotic coverage is started; a combination of penicillin and chloramphenicol is commonly used. Antibiotics alone may appear to produce a cure, but usually do not. Brain abscess usually requires surgery for definitive treatment. Most neurosurgeons recommend early operative drainage. Rupture of the abscess into the ventricles and transtentorial herniation are fatal complications. Later removal of the abscess cavity can be performed if it is accessible.

NOTE: When a child with congenital heart disease, chronic otitis, sinusitis, mastoiditis, or lung disease develops headache and/or neurologic signs and symptoms, a brain abscess must be ruled out.

Suggested Readings

Bell WE, McCormick WF: Neurologic Infections in Children, 2nd ed, vol XII of Major Problems in Clinical Pediatrics. Philadelphia, W.B. Saunders, 1981.

Dodge PR, Swartz MN: Bacterial meningitis - a review of selected aspects. N Engl J Med 272:725, 779, 842, 898, 954, 1003, 1965.

Feigin RD, Cherry JD: Textbook of Pediatric Infectious Diseases. Philadelphia, W.B. Saunders, 1981, pp 293–345, 754–755.

Horwitz SF, et al: Cerebral herniation in bacterial meningitis in childhood. Ann Neurol 7:524, 1980.

Matson DD: Neurosurgery of Infancy and Childhood, Springfield, IL, Charles C Thomas, 1969, pp 708–730.

Smith DH, Ingram DL, Smith AL, Gilles F, Bresnan MF: Bacterial meningitis, a symposium. Pediatrics 52:586, 1973.

Chapter 20

Metabolic and Toxic Encephalopathies

The term <u>toxic encephalopathy</u> has special meaning for pediatricians. It is often heralded by a febrile illness, depressed consciousness, and occasionally seizures. There usually is elevated cerebrospinal fluid (CSF) pressure without cells, sometimes a minimally increased protein, and a swollen brain without evidence of inflammation. In 1963 Reye and his colleagues defined a subgroup of these children based on abnormal liver function tests, hypoglycemia, and fatty infiltration of the liver. Since then Reye's syndrome is recognized as the most important identifiable group of toxic encephalopathies. Lead encephalopathy is also associated with raised intracranial pressure and brain swelling.

<u>Metabolic encephalopathies</u> in childhood represent the reaction of the central nervous system (CNS) to a specific metabolic derangement, e.g., hypoglycemia, diabetic coma, hyper- and hyponatremia, hypoxia, uremia, liver failure, and burns. Brain swelling <u>per se</u> is less clearly a problem. The treatment of metabolic encephalopathy is the treatment of the underlying metabolic derangement.

The differential diagnosis of a child with toxic or metabolic encephalopathy includes:

1. Ingestion.

2. Meningitis, acute and subacute.

3. Viral encephalitis.

4. Subdural hematoma.

5. Brain abscess.

6. Confusional migraine.

7. Petit mal status.

REYE'S SYNDROME

Clinical Picture

Characteristically, there is a preceding "flu-like" febrile illness that precedes the acute encephalopathy by 7 to 10 days. Influenza B is the "epidemic flu" most commonly associated with large outbreaks. Varicella is the exanthema most commonly associated with Reye's syndrome. As the child recovers from his illness, pernicious vomiting and lethargy develop. Liver function studies (ammonia and serum glutamic oxaloacetic transaminase (SGOT) levels) are abnormal (Stage I).

Disorientation, delirium (often with hallucinations), and combativeness follow; hyperventilation is prominent. The child becomes stuporous, i.e., he can be aroused by noxious stimuli and will respond appropriately by pushing the stimulus away. By this time, liver function studies are clearly abnormal (Stage II).

Now the child is critically ill and may rapidly become comatose with decortication (flexion of the upper extremities and hyperextension of the legs) and have bilateral upgoing toes (Stage III). Hyperventilation ("central," neurogenic) continues and seizures can occur which, in conjunction with cardiac or respiratory arrest, may herald the onset of decerebration (Stage IV). The child extends his upper extremities and intorts his legs to painful stimuli and occasionally spontaneously. Tone is increased and cranial nerve abnormalities, including abnormalities of ocular movements and pupil size, may occur.

Liver function tests may begin to return toward normal despite continuing decerebration.

In the final stage (V), the child becomes flaccid, all brainstem functions cease, and respiratory support is needed.

TABLE 20.1

REYE'S SYNDROME: DEGREE OF CLINICAL ABNORMALITY

Stage I	Vomiting, lethargy, drowsiness, extensor plantars with evidence of liver dysfunction
Stage II	Disorientation and combativeness, semicoma, hyperventilation, marked increase in liver dysfunction
Stage III	Coma, hyperventilation, upper midbrain dysfunction with decortication, continued liver function abnormalities
Stage IV	Deepening coma, lower midbrain dysfunction with decerebration, continued liver function abnormalities
Stage V	Coma, medullary involvement with respiratory arrest, even though improvement of liver dysfunction may occur

Laboratory

In addition to abnormal liver function tests there is a combined respiratory alkalosis and metabolic acidosis. Hypoglycemia occurs in younger children. Lumbar puncture may show an elevated CSF pressure without cells and normal protein. EEG changes are marked, and the EEG is a sensitive indicator of the level of CNS dysfunction.

Of all the chemical studies, the serum ammonia level is of greatest importance; an ammonia over 300 $\mu g/100$ ml carries a poor prognosis.

When a child presents in the acute phase, a lumbar puncture (LP) is often necessary to rule out meningitis. However, a lumbar puncture in the presence of increased intracranial pressure is potentially dangerous, and if the history is characteristic of Reye's syndrome and there is no nuchal rigidity, it is best to wait for the results of liver function studies (SGOT, NH$_3$); if they are elevated, an LP is not performed.

Treatment

Modes of therapy recommended combine careful metabolic management and measures to monitor and combat cerebral edema. These latter include mannitol (6 gm/kg/day), glycerol (6 gm/kg/day), and fluid restriction to 40 ml/kg/day. Treatment requires a multidisciplinary intensive care team.

Prognosis

Initial mortality figures from retrospective studies ranged from 80 to 100%. As Reye's syndrome has become increasingly recognized, this figure has dropped to less than 30%. The more rapid the progression through the various stages, the poorer the prognosis.

Factors associated with a poor prognosis:

1. Ammonia greater than 300 $\mu g/100$ ml.

2. Very rapid progression through early stages.

3. Elevated CSF pressure (no tap).

4. Grade 3 EEG.

5. Seizures.

Complete recovery is probable from Stages I through III. Recovery from Stage IV occurs only with vigorous therapy and some survivors may have residual CNS damage.

LEAD ENCEPHALOPATHY

Lead is an important cause of toxic encephalopathy. The clinical picture includes ataxia, lethargy, coma, and seizures. There may be raised intracranial pressure with papilledema and split sutures on skull x-ray. Usually there are few focal signs. A high index of suspicion is the cornerstone for diagnosis. Diagnosis ultimately depends on blood and/or urine lead levels, but may be suspected on the basis of hematologic (free erythrocyte porphyrin (FEP)) and radiologic abnormalities. LP is contraindicated in children with lead encephalopathy; raised intracranial pressure is treated with dexamethasone and osmotic agents (see Chap. 22). Seizures are treated with standard anticonvulsants but may be difficult to control.

Treatment

(1) EDTA, 50 to 75 mg/kg i.v. or i.m. in three divided doses per day for 5 days, repeat as necessary. Check urine for WBC's and follow blood urea nigrogen (BUN) and creatinine for evidence of renal tubular injury. (2) Dimercaprol (BAL), 12 to 24 mg/kg i.m. for 24 hours in three divided doses per day for 5 days, if there is evidence of encephalopathy or the blood lead is greater than 100 μg/100 ml. (3) Cathartics, if gut films are positive for lead. (4) D-Penicillamine, 20 to 40 mg/kg orally per day for long term management. (5) Remember, prevention involves ensuring a lead-free environment.

Classical severe lead encephalopathy seems to be occurring less frequently; however, there is increasing concern about low level exposure and increased lead burden (blood level 30 to 60 μg/ml, FEP 100 μg/100 ml, 24-hour urinary lead excretion 80 to 100 μg) and its potential effect on the CNS.

Suggested Readings

Boutros, AR: Reye syndrome: a predictably curable disease. Pediatr Clin North Am 27:539, 1980.
Needleman HL: Low Level Lead Exposure. New York, Raven Press, 1980.
Shaywitz BA, et al: Monitoring and management of increased intracranial pressure in Reye syndrome: results in 29 children. Pediatrics 66:198, 1980.
Trauner, DA: Treatment of Reye syndrome. Ann Neurol 7:2, 1980.

Chapter 21

Lumbar Puncture

INDICATIONS

1. When central nervous system (CNS) infection is
    suspected one must examine the cerebrospinal fluid
    (CSF). (Exception: if one suspects brain abscess or
    other significant mass lesion, CAT scan and neurologic
    consultation are needed.) An LP may be performed to
    establish CSF bleeding -- e.g., intraventricular or
    subarachnoid hemorrhage, although bleeding is usually
    visible on CAT scan.

2. An LP is performed when CSF chemistries have
    diagnostic value -- e.g., gamma-globulin and measles
    antibody in suspected SSPE and elevated protein in
    polyneuritis.

3. Lumbar puncture is needed for the study of CSF
    dynamics -- e.g., when checking for spinal block,
    though radiologic and neurosurgical standby is
    critical when these studies are performed.

4. Therapeutically, an LP may be done to inject
    methotrexate for CNS leukemia or amphotericin B for
    fungal meningitis, to remove fluid as treatment for
    benign raised intracranial pressure (pseudotumor
    cerebri), or for the headache of subarachnoid
    hemorrhage.

CONTRAINDICATIONS

1. Infection at the site of the lumbar puncture.

2. When a cerebral mass lesion is suspected, particularly in a child with lateralized neurologic signs.

   Brain abscesses (usually seen in congenital heart disease with right-to-left shunts, otitis media, or lung disease) may produce transtentorial herniation after LP.

   Brain tumors may lead to herniation, especially when in the posterior fossa.

   Subdural hematoma is not usually diagnosed by LP and the removal of spinal fluid may be harmful.

   In these instances, a search for a mass lesion via CAT scan or MRI should be done before the LP. If a focal lesion or shift of midline is discovered, one would not perform an LP.

3. Lumbar puncture should not be done in the presence of papilledema (a check of the fundi must precede each LP). An LP may ultimately be done in a child with papilledema (if CSF examination is crucial), but only after neurologic and/or neurosurgical consultation.

4. Lumbar puncture is probably harmful in children with Reye's syndrome and lead encephalopathy because of cerebral edema associated with these entities.

5. If a spinal block is suspected, an LP should be done in a situation where contrast dye can be injected if necessary without withdrawing the needle. Neurosurgical backup should be available, as an LP with fluid removal can convert a partial block to a complete one.

COMPLICATIONS

   Post-LP headache rarely occurs in children; it is common in adults and may be seen in adolescents. It is characteristically exacerbated by sitting or standing and relieved by lying flat. It is seen within the first 1 to 3 days after the LP; it usually lasts 2 to 5 days although it may persist for weeks. Treatment consists of bed rest and fluids. Post-LP headache may be minimized by using a small gauge needle and removing a minimal amount of fluid.

Occasionally there will be some paraspinal muscle spasm and even more rarely sciatic pain related to a nerve root being caught by the LP needle. This may lead to a brief reluctance to walk by some children.

When there is an unexpected raised pressure (it must stay elevated after the child has relaxed with legs extended or has stopped crying and the head is no longer flexed), remove minimal fluid needed for studies. Neurologic and/or neurosurgical consultation should be obtained and the child watched carefully over the ensuing hours for signs of deterioration. Children with meningitis may have markedly elevated pressures, but these pressures are not as dangerous as raised intracranial pressure secondary to focal lesion. Remember, hypercarbia, water intoxication, and hypertensive encephalopathy (acute glomerulonephritis) are remediable causes of raised intracranial pressure. When the intracranial pressure is raised and there is neurologic deterioration immediately or during the hours after the LP, treatment with osmotic dehydrating agents and steroids is indicated (see Chap. 22).

If the child has a partial or almost complete spinal block secondary to compression of the cord (e.g., by tumor) CSF removal may cause rapid worsening of the block. Signs of block include abnormal manometric findings and xanthochromatic fluid under low pressure (see Chap. 14 for treatment). Do not remove the needle if this is found; the needle can be used to instill appropriate dye to myelography.

The practice of performing an LP in the neonate without a stylet carries the rare potential danger of introducing a pledget of skin, which may subsequently lead to the development of a dermoid.

METHOD OF LUMBAR PUNCTURE

1. The puncture is carried out between L4-5 located by the level of iliac crest; the L5-S1 interspace may also be used.

2. Inset the bevel of the needle parallel to the long axis of the spine.

3. If manometric studies and myelography are not being
    performed, use a 22-gauge needle.

4. Note the opening and closing pressure as well as the
    amount of fluid removed.

    //Accurate pressure recording is an integral
         part of a well performed LP.//

5. Coughing, crying, or abdominal pressure cause delayed
    venous return around the cord and should increase CSF
    flow and pressure. These maneuvers show that the
    needle is in place, but they do not test for spinal
    subarachnoid block. For this, manometric studies are
    performed (jugular pressure is raised via hand
    pressure around the neck) and the rise and fall of CSF
    pressure are recorded. Manometric studies are not
    done routinely and never if the baseline pressure is
    elevated or an intracranial lesion is suspected.

6. Proper positioning of the child is crucial for
    successful lumbar puncture; thus, the person holding
    the child is often as important as the person
    performing the LP.

    //Positioning is crucial for a successful LP.//

    The child should be placed in the fetal position with
    the back at right angles to the bed. In some
    children, sedation may be of value. Insert the needle
    under the skin (after local anesthesia) and then
    decide on the angle of entry. Make sure the needle is
    strictly parallel to the bed and angled toward the
    child's umbilicus. Once the needle has been advanced,
    if it does not enter the subarachnoid space or
    encounters bone, the direction of the needle cannot be
    changed. Pull the needle back to just beneath the
    skin and redirect it. With experience one will learn
    to recognize the familiar "pop" as the needle enters
    the subarachnoid space. If the LP is not possible in
    the fetal position, have the child sit up and lean
    forward grasping a pillow; try again in the sitting
    position (it is easier to gauge the midline).
    Remember, sitting pressures are unreliable.

7. When an LP is impossible because of bony anomalies or
    local infection, and CSF examination is crucial, one
    should arrange for cisternal tap or an LP done under
    fluoroscopy.

EXAMINATION OF THE CSF

The Fluid

1. Collect Five Tubes: the first is used to look for cells, the second is for bacteriologic studies, the third tube is for chemistry studies (protein and glucose), the fourth tube is for a cell count by the physician (particularly useful in circumstances of traumatic puncture), and the fifth tube may be saved and used for cytologic investigation if appropriate. (A sample may be lost, an unexpected chemistry value return demanding a repeat determination, or a new test wanted.) If there is the possibility of a traumatic tap, cells are counted in both the first and third tubes.

2. If red blood cells (RBCs) are present, count them in the first and third tubes. In subarachnoid or intracranial bleeding, the amount of blood remains constant in each tube, and the blood does not clot. Decreasing numbers of cells suggest a traumatic tap. After centrifugation, the CSF from a traumatic tap will be clear while with true CNS bleeding the supernatant is xanthochromatic if the bleeding occurred at least 2 to 4 hours previously. Finding crenated RBCs is of no value as they appear both with true bleeding and after traumatic taps.

3. Check to see if the CSF is clear by comparing it with water. A CSF protein greater than 100 mg/100 ml usually causes the spinal fluid to look faintly yellow. Approximately 200 to 300 white blood cells (WBCs) are needed to cause CSF cloudiness. Subdural hematoma and jaundice may produce xanthochromia.

4. Always examine the CSF for cells within 1 hour after LP and preferably sooner. Normally there should be no polymorphonuclear neutrophils (PMNs) and no more than 3 to 5 lymphocytes. Up to 10 cells in the first 3 days of life is sufficiently common to be considered "normal," including one or two PMNs. It is very important to distinguish between RBCs and WBCs. After a total cell count is done, add acetic acid to the spinal fluid; this lyses the RBCs, but leaves the WBCs intact. (Rinse a capillary tube with acetic acid and then draw the CSF into the tube.) Often one can distinguish between PMNs and lymphocytes by adding methylene blue to the fluid. When looking for tumor

cells, or if the nature of the WBCs in the CSF is questioned, a Millipore or cytologic (e.g., cytocentrifuge) examination is indicated. When bacterial or tuberculous infection is suspected, perform a Gram stain or acid fast stain on the centrifuged sediment; when fungal disease is a possibility, do an India ink preparation. (Place a coverslip over 1 drop of CSF on a slide. Place a drop if India ink next to the coverslip and allow it to seep under. Check at the interface for <u>Cryptococcus</u>.)

5. When there are RBCs in the CSF and the child has a normal CBC, expect one WBC for every 700 RBCs (make further corrections for anemia or leukocytosis). In addition, every 700 RBCs raise the protein by 1 mg/100 ml.

INTERPRETATION

<u>Glucose</u> (normal CSF glucose is two-thirds blood glucose).

<u>Increased</u> glucose levels are not significant, they reflect systemic hyperglycemia. With changing blood glucose, CSF glucose lags behind blood glucose by approximately 1 hour. With systemic hyperglycemia, a concomitant blood glucose is needed to demonstrate a relatively lowered CSF glucose that might otherwise be considered normal.

<u>Decreased</u> glucose levels are seen in bacterial, tuberculous, and fungal meningitis and sometimes with meningeal involvement by neoplasm or a nontuberculous granulomatous process such as sarcoidosis. Although characteristically normal in viral infections, the CSF glucose has been reported low with certain CNS viral infections (herpes, mumps, and lymphocytic choriomeningitis). Decreased CSF glucose is secondary to changes in carbohydrate metabolism by adjacent tissue, WBC utilization of glucose, and alteration of glucose transport into the CNS.

<u>Protein</u>

Protein levels are increased in a wide variety of neurologic diseases and usually reflect an abnormality in the blood-brain barrier. Elevated levels are seen in processes affecting nerve roots in peripheral neuropathy. Normal CSF protein is less than 40 mg/100 ml in children older than 1 month. In fact, most children have a protein less than 30 mg/100 ml. Until 1 month of age, a level of less than 100 mg/100 ml is normal.

1. Brain tumor frequently produces a protein elevation of 100 to 200 mg/100 ml, although the level may be normal. CSF protein in brainstem gliomas is generally normal.

2. Spinal cord tumors raise CSF protein, often to extremely high levels (e.g., 750 to 1000 mg/100 ml), especially when block is present.

3. Purulent meningitis elevates the protein level regardless of the cause. Viral infections of the CNS are associated with normal or mild increases in protein.

4. Infectious polyneuritis (Guillain-Barre syndrome) characteristically causes increased protein levels. The protein may be normal during the first few days of the illness but rises after 7 to 14 days.

5. Degenerative disease may show elevated CSF protein -- metachromatic leukodystrophy, Krabbe's disease.

6. Lead intoxication typically has an elevated protein (remember, LP is hazardous in lead encephalopathy).

Colloidal Gold Reaction

This reaction depends on the ratio of albumin to gamma-globulin. Its sensitivity varies greatly and it has been replaced by actual measurements of albumin and gamma-globulin. Do not waste fluid if gamma-globulin levels are available.

Gamma-Globulin

Normally, gamma-globulin represents 15% or less of the total protein. (If total protein values are less than 20 mg/100 ml, the percentage of gamma-globulin may be unreliable.) Gamma-globulin is dramatically elevated in subacute sclerosing panencephalitis and may be elevated in multiple sclerosis, Schilder's disease, and herpes encephalitis. Oligoclonal banding studies of CSF protein may be useful in determining the origin of the elevated protein production.

CSF Pressure

The CSF pressure is normally less than 180 mm H_2O. In neonates it is less than 100 mm H_2O. It is not affected by changes in systemic arterial blood pressure but is exquisitely sensitive to changes in blood CO_2 (hyperventilation lowers intracranial pressure) and venous pressure.

1. Elevated pressures are seen in acute bacterial, fungal, and viral meningitis or meningoencephalitis.

2. There frequently is elevation with tumors or other intracerebral mass lesions, although pressure may be normal despite a large tumor.

3. Pressure is usually elevated in intracerebral bleeding and in subarachnoid hemorrhage.

4. The pressure and protein may be raised and there may be papilledema with polyneuritis or spinal tumor.

5. Unexplained elevated pressures may be due to congestive heart failure, pulmonary disease with hypercapnia, jugular venous obstruction, or pericardial effusion; increases are also seen with most general anesthetics.

6. Pseudotumor cerebri (benign raised intracranial pressure, benign intracranial hypertension: BIH) refers to raised pressure (as high as 400 to 600 mm H_2O) with papilledema, not associated with a mass lesion or hydrocephalus, and with otherwise normal CSF. These children are relatively asymptomatic apart from headache and, at times, diplopia (usually related to sixth nerve palsy) or blurred vision. Causes include lateral venous sinus occlusion secondary to otitis, withdrawal from steroids, head trauma, topical steroids, pregnancy, oral contraceptives, hypo- or hypervitaminosis A, hypoparathyroidism, and tetracycline administration. Often the process is idiopathic. One must first rule out tumor and hydrocephalus with CAT scan. Then the diagnosis can be established by LP. Lumbar punctures alone are often sufficient to lower CSF pressure and reverse the process. Acetazolamide may be given to decrease CSF production. Oral glycerol and steroids (see Chap. 22) can be used if needed. Visual difficulties and actual loss of vision occur and warrant vigorous treatment

with frequent LPs in addition to steroids and
acetazolamide. Rarely, a lumboperitoneal shunt will
be required.

Pleocytosis

PMNs in the CSF suggest a bacterial infection, and
lymphocytes suggest a viral or chronic inflammatory
process (although PMNs are often seen at the onset of a
viral process). WBCs may be seen after subarachnoid
hemorrhage, thrombosis, and, at times, with tumor.
Atypical lymphocytes are present with infectious
mononucleosis; eosinophils suggest a parasitic infection
or dye reaction. Remember, many organic diseases of the
CNS produce a mild pleocytosis. A thorough bacteriologic
investigation must be carried out in all instances, even
though cells do not always represent infection. Red cells
usually represent intracranial bleeding or a traumatic
lumbar puncture.

Suggested Readings

Bell WE, McCormick WF: Increased Intracranial
Pressure in Children, ed 2, vol 8 of Major Problems in
Clinical Pediatrics. Philadelphia, W.B. Saunders, 1977.
Fishman RA: Cerebrospinal Fluid in Diseases of the
Nervous System. Philadelphia, W.B. Saunders, 1980.
Weisberg LA, Chutorian AM: Pseudotumor cerebri of
childhood. Am J Dis Child 131:1243, 1977.

Chapter 22

Raised Intracranial Pressure

AGENTS USED IN TREATING INTRACRANIAL PRESSURE

Hyperventilation

Hyperventilation may be used in acute situations (e.g., head trauma, toxic encephalopathy) and is sometimes employed during neurosurgical procedures. By lowering the PCO_2 to 25 to 30 mm Hg, there is reduced cerebral blood flow and an immediate reduction of intracranial pressure. Do not lower PCO_2 below 25 mm Hg as it may be harmful, significantly decreasing cerebral blood flow. If a child is brought to the emergency ward after severe head trauma and clinical deterioration is rapid, intubation and hyperventilation are effective means of lowering the pressure until such agents as mannitol take effect and neurosurgery or other treatment is instituted.

Mannitol

Mannitol, an osmotic dehydrating agent, crosses the blood-brain barrier slowly, and because it is hypertonic, draws intracerebral water into the intravascular space. It is given at a dose of 0.5 to 1.0 gm/kg i.v. over 5 to 10 minutes and 0.5 to 1.0 gm/kg i.v. every 6 hours. It is usually not given for more than 24 to 48 hours and is used in acute situations to "buy time" (e.g., after head trauma or deterioration from an expanding intracranial process), often prior to neurosurgical intervention. The onset of action is approximately 15 minutes. Urea is similar to mannitol in its use, mode of action, and dose (1 gm/kg) but is given most often by nasogastric tube. These agents must be given with caution to children who have renal or cardiac disease. There may be "rebound" after their use (viz., return of water intracerebrally). Remember to catheterize the comatose child given osmotic agents.

Steroids

Steroids (dexamethasone) are used both acutely and chronically (give 0.2 mg/kg i.v. as initial dose, then 0.5 mg/kg/day i.v., i.m., or p.o. in four divided doses). The onset of action is approximately 12 to 24 hours. Dexamethasone is given in acute situations and may become the mainstay of treatment after 12 to 24 hours. It is used palliatively to treat brain tumor, after neurosurgical procedures, and sometimes concomitantly with radiation therapy to the brain. The mechanism of steroid action is poorly understood.

Glycerol

Glycerol, an osmotic dehydrating agent, is slower acting than mannitol/urea (onset of action is approximately 12 hours) but can be used for longer periods of time. It is given orally in a dose of 0.5 to 1 gm/kg every 6 hours; it may be given via nasogastric tube, and some have used it intravenously. It does not have the potential side effects of prolonged steroid administration, and there is little "rebound" after its use. Glycerol is used to treat swelling associated with toxic encephalopathies and after neurosurgical procedures or trauma, and it can be used concomitantly with steroids.

Ventricular Puncture

Ventricular puncture or surgical decompression may be carried out when mechanical release of raised intracranial pressure is needed. However, when the pressure is due to intraparenchymal disease rather than to a block and hydrocephalus, puncturing the ventricles can be both difficult and hazardous.

Treatment

Transtentorial herniation secondary to increased intracranial pressure caused by supratentorial lesions (e.g., subdural hematoma, intracerebral hemorrhage) often presents a recognizable clinical syndrome. Transtentorial herniation is a neurologic emergency; mannitol should be given immediately and neurosurgical consultation obtained. After mannitol administration, 0.2 mg/kg of dexamethasone should be given and, if clinically appropriate, intubation and hyperventilation begun.

HERNIATION SYNDROMES

There are two clinical syndromes of transtentorial herniation; these syndromes represent loss of neurologic function that begins in the cerebral hemispheres and progresses to involve upper then lower brainstem with death the end result.

A. Uncal (Lateral) Syndrome of Herniation

1. A unilaterally dilated pupil is the first sign secondary to a mass in the middle fossa (e.g., temporal lobe) pushing the uncus medially and trapping the third nerve. A contralateral hemiplegia is usually present. Initially, respiration and consciousness are unimpaired.

2. Progressive pressure leads to increasing stupor, a more complete third nerve palsy, and often an ipsilateral hemiplegia with bilateral Babinski responses. The ipsilateral hemiplegia is secondary to the opposite cerebral peduncle being pushed against the tentorium (Kernohan's notch). Respiration may be normal or of the central neurogenic hyperventilation pattern. There is often decerebrate posturing (arms extended at the side with inward turning either spontaneously or when a noxious stimulus is applied). Decorticate posturing (arms flexed at the elbow, "pointing" to the cortex) is not usually seen with the uncal syndrome.

3. Further pressure leads to prominent brainstem dysfunction with dilation of both pupils, loss of brainstem reflexes (e.g., absent doll's eyes maneuver, no response to ice-water calorics), ataxic respiratory patterns, and bilateral decerebrate rigidity. Treatment at this stage is rarely of benefit.

B. Central Syndrome of Herniation

1. Pressure is exerted centrally on the diencephalon, rather than laterally as occurs in the uncal syndrome. The first sign is a change in alertness or behavior. Respiration is usually normal or contains frequent

sighs or yawns. Brainstem function is intact though pupils are small and there may be roving eye movements. There usually are Babinski responses, and there may be rigidity of the extremities. With progression there is decorticate posturing.

2. Involvement of upper brainstem leads to dilation of both pupils and impairment of oculovestibular reflexes (e.g., absent or abnormal doll's eyes maneuver). Central neurogenic hyperventilation often occurs and decorticate posturing progresses to decerebrate posturing. There may be wide fluctuations in body temperature.

3. Further progression leads to loss of all brainstem function with ataxic breathing, then apnea and death.

These syndromes can progress over hours or may occur in minutes, depending on the pathologic process. The uncal syndrome is typically seen secondary to space occupying lesions, such as intracranial hemorrhage or brain abscess. The central syndrome is usually seen with diffuse increased intracranial pressure, e.g., Reye's syndrome, acute hydrocephalus.

Suggested Readings

Bell WE, McCormick WF: Increased Intracranial Pressure in Children, vol. 8 of Major Problems in Clinical Pedriatrics. Philadelphia, W.B. Saunders, 1978.
Miller JD: Barbiturates and raised intracranial pressure. Ann Neurol 6:189, 1979.
Plum F, Posner JB: Diagnosis of Stupor and Coma, 3rd ed. Philadelphia, F.A. Davis, 1980.

Chapter 23

Head Trauma

Head injury is a dynamic process. Parameters to monitor are the child's level of consciousness and mental status. Important guidelines in dealing with the child are:

1. In <u>severe head trauma</u>, control of airway and intravenous line placement are first priorities. One should assume the child has a fractured cervical spine and avoid turning the head; obtain cervical spine films in addition to skull x-rays. Look for accompanying traumatic injury to abdominal and thoracic organs. If a child has head injury and shock, assume they are unrelated.

2. In all cases of head trauma, <u>neurologic examination</u> should be performed and must <u>include (a) careful</u> documentation of the child's level of consciousness and ability to carry out mental tasks appropriate for age; (b) a careful look at the tympanic membranes for evidence of basilar skull fracture (blood or CSF); (c) scalp examination for evidence of localized areas of trauma; a bruise over the mastoid (Battle's sign) is indicative of a fracture; (d) precise recording of pupillary size and reaction; monitor heart rate, blood pressure, and respiratory pattern (a slow pulse and high blood pressure indicate raised intracranial pressure); (e) check for hemiparesis and presence or absence of upgoing toes; and (f) measure head circumference in infants and toddlers with head trauma.

3. Concussion is defined as an immediate and transient loss of consciousness following head injury. There may be amnesia for events that occurred prior to and after the head injury.

4. Observation in the hospital for a period of 24 to 48 hours and neurosurgical consultation are appropriate for a child with any focal abnormalities on neurologic examination, an abnormal mental status, skull fracture, or head trauma that is believed to be significant despite a normal examination. The decision to hospitalize or send home a child who has had a period of unconsciousness and who has a normal neurologic examination must be made on the basis of who will look after him.

5. One of the most feared complications of head injury is the development of a subdural or epidural hematoma and subsequent fatal brainstem compression. Clinically, this process manifests itself as headache, decreased level of consciousness, and, late in the course, a dilated pupil on the side of the hematoma secondary to pressure on the third nerve. Epidural hematoma represents (a) venous bleeding or (b) arterial bleeding secondary to a tear in the middle meningeal artery. The child may steadily deteriorate following the trauma or experience a "lucid interval" only to deteriorate later. Older children may or may not have a fracture line over the groove of the middle meningeal artery. Subdural hematoma represents venous or arterial bleeding and similarly has the potential for brainstem compression. Remember, subdural hematomas can occur in the posterior fossa, producing gait difficulties. These may be associated with linear occipital fractures, especially those traversing a sinus groove.

6. We feel there is potential danger and no value in performing a lumbar puncture in a child with head trauma.

7. Skull films are an important part of the evaluation of a child with head trauma and loss of consciousness despite the small percentage that show an abnormality. When the following signs and/or symptoms are present, there is a high yield of positive findings on skull x-ray: (a) loss of consciousness or amnesia greater than 5 minutes; (b) vomiting; (c) discharge from the ear or nose, discolored eardrum; (d) bilateral black

eyes; (e) lethargy or stupor; (f) focal neurologic signs, including anisocoria, focal weakness, or Babinski response.

8. The battered child syndrome is always a consideration when the extent of the injury seems excessive or unexplained by the clinical story.

9. Transient blindness or sixth nerve palsies after head trauma are not uncommon in children. Fortunately, these children invariably recover.

Suggested Readings

Brink JD, et al: Physical recovery after severe closed head trauma in children and adolescents. J Pediatr 97:721, 1980.

Raphaely RC, et al: Management of severe pediatric head trauma. Pediatr Clin North Am 27:715, 1980.

Rosman NP, et al: Acute head trauma in infancy and childhood. Pediatr Clin North Am 26:707, 1979.

Chapter 24

Neurocutaneous Syndromes (Phakomatoses)

The neurocutaneous syndromes include a group of developmental disorders that affect both skin and nervous system and have a high association with tumors and congenital malformations. A complete listing would include over 25 entities; the more common syndromes are discussed below.

NEUROFIBROMATOSIS (VON RECKLINGHAUSEN'S DISEASE)

The characteristic cutaneous manifestations of neurofibromatosis are yellow-brown cafe-au-lait spots and cutaneous neurofibromas. A diagnosis can be made on the basis of five or more spots that exceed 1.5 cm in diameter in teenagers or 0.5 cm in young children. Only 1 to 2% of normal controls have more than two cafe-au-lait spots. Cafe-au-lait spots may be present at birth or appear during the 1st or 2nd decade. Neurofibromas are usually multiple, are of varied size, and are either cutaneous or attached to subcutaneous nerve trunks; they are rarely painful. Axillary freckling is highly associated with neurofibromatosis. Inheritance is autosomal dominant, but there is a high mutation rate.

Neurologically, these children are at increased risk to develop tumors (often multiple) in both the central and peripheral nervous systems: optic nerve gliomas, bilateral acoustic neuromas, astrocytomas, meningiomas, and tumors compressing the spinal cord. Intracranial tumors may be associated with seizures; mental retardation is uncommon in children with neurofibromatosis, but the frequency of less than average intelligence is high. Involvement of adrenals (pheochromocytoma) and other endocrine glands, renal artery stenosis (high blood pressure), skeletal abnormalities, and thoracic and abdominal tumors are also seen in von Recklinghausen's disease.

TUBEROUS SCLEROSIS

The classic triad of tuberous sclerosis is adenoma sebaceum, mental retardation, and epilepsy. Adenoma sebaceum consists of a nodular or papular erythematous rash found in a butterfly pattern across the nose, cheek, and in the nasolabial fold. It is present in 80 to 90% of children with tuberous sclerosis, usually appears in early childhood, and may occur in intellectually normal affected individuals. Other cutaneous manifestations include shagreen patches (raised plaques found most commonly in the lumbar region), white, leaf-shaped macules (often present at birth and seen best with a Wood's light), cafe-au-lait spots, subungual fibromas, and gingival fibroma. The characteristic ophthalmologic finding is a light-colored nodule of the retina. Inheritance is autosomal dominant, although sporadic cases occur.

Neurologically, seizures and mental retardation are common, although children and adults may have cutaneous manifestations and no neurologic dysfunction. Tuberous sclerosis may present as infantile spasms; there is no specific treatment for children with tuberous sclerosis apart from control of the seizure disorder with anticonvulsants. Pathologic findings include tubers of the cerebral cortex, intraventricular tumors (foramen of Monro), and an increased incidence of parenchymal brain tumors. There may be tumors of other organs, including kidney (in over two-thirds of cases), heart, and abdominal viscera. Calcifications on CAT scan are evident early, often in the 1st year of life. Skull x-rays show calcification much later and with less frequency.

STURGE-WEBER SYNDROME (ENCEPHALOTRIGEMINAL ANGIOMATOSIS)

The characteristic features of this disorder are a port wine stain involving the face (usually in the distribution of the first division of the trigeminal nerve, i.e., forehead) and an ipsilateral (or bilateral) vascular malformation of the parietal-occipital meninges overlying an ischemic atrophic cerebral cortex. Calcification of underlying gyri develops during infancy and gives a unique "railroad track" appearance on skull x-ray. CAT scan may show changes earlier than can be demonstrated by skull x-ray or even angiography. These children have a tendency to develop glaucoma on the affected side (buphthalmos) and often have a contralateral hemiplegia and hemianopsia, seizure disorder, and mental retardation. Treatment involves anticonvulsants, monitoring for glaucoma, and sometimes attempts at surgical removal of the malformation.

VON HIPPEL-LINDAU DISEASE (ANGIOMATOSIS OF THE RETINA AND CEREBELLUM)

This autosomal dominant disorder is characterized by an association between retinal and cerebellar angiomas. Tumors of the kidney and pancreas and an elevated hematocrit secondary to erythropoietin produced by the cerebellar tumor occur. Clinically, there are signs and symptoms of a posterior fossa tumor (ataxia, headache, and papilledema); treatment is surgical. Vascular malformations of the brainstem and spinal cord may also be associated with retinal angiomas (Wyburn-Mason syndrome).

Suggested readings

Chalhub EG: The neurocutaneous syndromes in children. Pediatr Clin North Amer 23:449, 1976.

Gomez MR: Tuberous Sclerosis. New York, Raven Press, 1979.

Riccardi VM: Von Recklinghausen neurofibromatosis. N Engl J Med 305:1617, 1981.

Chapter 25

Neuroanatomy

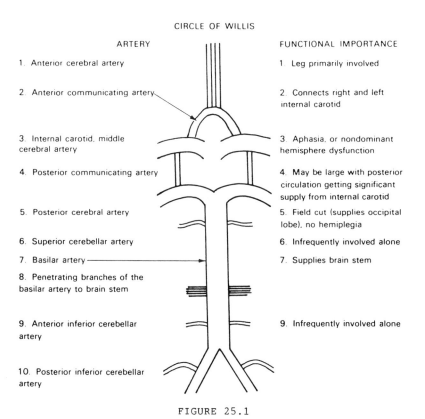

CIRCLE OF WILLIS

ARTERY	FUNCTIONAL IMPORTANCE
1. Anterior cerebral artery	1. Leg primarily involved
2. Anterior communicating artery	2. Connects right and left internal carotid
3. Internal carotid, middle cerebral artery	3. Aphasia, or nondominant hemisphere dysfunction
4. Posterior communicating artery	4. May be large with posterior circulation getting significant supply from internal carotid
5. Posterior cerebral artery	5. Field cut (supplies occipital lobe), no hemiplegia
6. Superior cerebellar artery	6. Infrequently involved alone
7. Basilar artery	7. Supplies brain stem
8. Penetrating branches of the basilar artery to brain stem	
9. Anterior inferior cerebellar artery	9. Infrequently involved alone
10. Posterior inferior cerebellar artery	

FIGURE 25.1

EYE DEVIATION IN NEUROLOGIC DISEASE

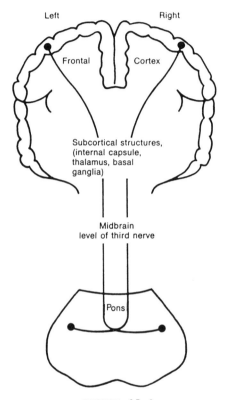

FIGURE 25.2

NOTE: the frontal eye fields exert a major
influence on horizontal eye movement, each field being
concerned with contralateral eye deviation. Thus, the
right field causes eyes to move to the left. The fibers
cross in the pons and there connect to the extraocular
muscles via the medial longitudinal fasciculus and sixth
cranial nerve (see Fig. 25.3). Both fields are constantly
active, striking a balance; thus when one is more or less
active than the other, horizontal eye deviation results.

EYE DEVIATION

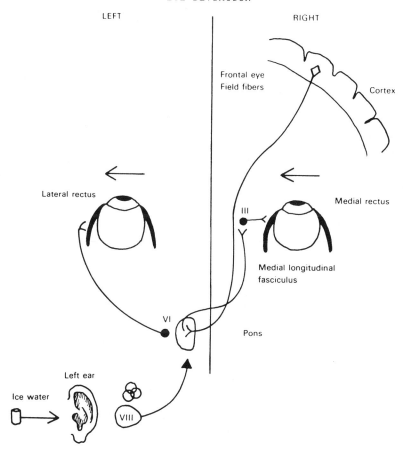

LEFT

RIGHT

Frontal eye
Field fibers

Cortex

Lateral rectus

Medial rectus

III

Medial longitudinal
fasciculus

VI

Pons

Left ear

Ice water

VIII

FIGURE 25.3

In the comatose child, ice water in the left ear
causes deviation of the eyes to the left. In the awake
child, this deviation is counteracted voluntarily,
producing nystagmus to the right.

A <u>destructive</u> <u>lesion</u> in the hemisphere or subcortex causes eyes to deviate toward the same side as the lesion. Thus, with a right-sided lesion the eyes are deviated to the right. An <u>excitatory</u> <u>lesion</u> at the cortical level (viz., a seizure) causes eyes to deviate to the contralateral side. Thus, with a left-sided seizure eyes are driven to the right. A <u>destructive</u> <u>lesion</u> in the pons (after fibers have crossed) causes eyes to deviate to the side opposite the damage. Thus, with a left-sided lesion eyes deviate to the right. (There are no excitatory lesions of the pons.) Eye deviation secondary to hemisphere lesions but not brainstem lesions may be overcome by brainstem reflexes, e.g., doll's eyes maneuver.

VISUAL PATHWAY

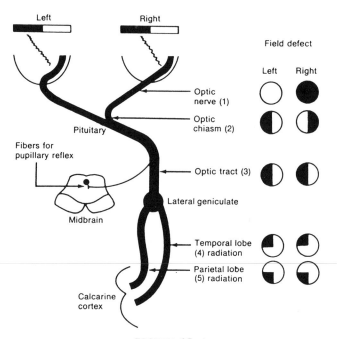

FIGURE 25.4

1. Blindness in one eye represents retinal or optic nerve dysfunction. The optic nerve is involved in optic neuritis, producing unilateral blindness; it may also be involved by tumor (optic glioma) or undergo atrophy secondary to prolonged raised intracranial pressure.

2. Bitemporal hemianopsia is classically found in craniopharyngiomas or pituitary tumors secondary to pressure on the optic chiasm. Nonhomonymous field defects usually imply a chiasmal lesion. Concentric "tunnel-like" vision may be seen in hysterical blindness.

3. Homonymous hemianopsia implies a lesion posterior to the chiasm. It may involve optic tract or both optic radiations emanating from the lateral geniculate body (or the lateral geniculate itself). The closer a lesion is to the lateral geniculate, the smaller it can be and still produce a homonymous hemianopsia.

4. The optic radiations fan out from the lateral geniculate and travel in the temporal and parietal lobes before reaching their destination in the occipital lobe. Lesions in the temporal lobe may give a homonymous superior field defect if the optic radiations are affected. Similarly, a lesion in the parietal lobe may show an inferior homonymous field defect.

5. The pupillary response is affected only if fibers proximal to the lateral geniculate body, in the midbrain, or third nerve are damaged.

6. When one realizes the enormous amount of territory needed for intact visual fields, it becomes apparent why checking visual fields is a mandatory part of every neurologic examination. In the infant, testing is often best done from behind, introducing objects into each lateral field individually and simultaneously. In young children ask them to look at your tongue, then wiggle a finger in the lateral field. If they see the fingers, they will automatically look at them.

SPINAL CORD

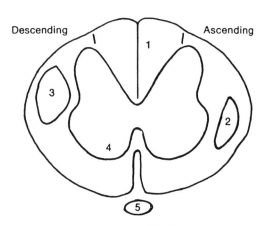

FIGURE 25.5

ASCENDING TRACTS

Dorsal columns (1) carry position and vibratory sense; fibers rise ipsilaterally and cross in the medulla. These columns are laminated, but the lamination is of no clinical importance.

Lateral spinothalamic tract (2) carries pain and temperature sensation. These fibers cross upon entering the cord; a cord lesion affecting them produces a contralateral loss. They are laminated with sacral fibers most laterally placed. Thus, an expanding process in the center of the cord gives sacral sparing (pinprick and temperature sensory loss are least prominent sacrally).

DESCENDING TRACTS

Lateral corticospinal tract (3) carries motor fibers and synapses in the anterior horn cells. The fibers have already crossed in the medulla. A lesion of, or pressure upon the corticospinal tract causes weakness, spasticity, hyperreflexia, and an upgoing toe.

Anterior horn cells (4) are lower motor neurons. A lesion here produces weakness, muscle wasting, fasciculations, and loss of reflexes.

VASCULAR SUPPLY

The <u>anterior</u> <u>spinal</u> <u>artery</u> (5) supplies the entire cord except for the dorsal columns. Thus, the anterior spinal artery syndrome produces paralysis and loss of pain and temperature sense; position and vibratory sense are preserved.

CLINICAL CORRELATION

. Friedreich's ataxia affects 1 and 3.

. Familial spastic paraplegia affects 3.

. Poliomyelitis and Werdnig-Hoffman disease affect 4.

. Brown-Sequard syndrome (hemisection of cord) produces ipsilateral paralysis and contralateral loss of sensation to pinprick.

MEDULLA (Cranial Nerves 9 to 12)

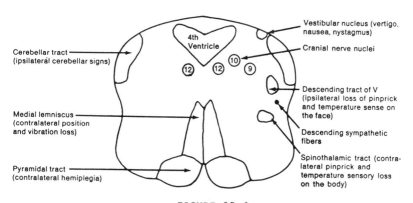

FIGURE 25.6

Remember that the <u>seventh</u> (facial) <u>nerve</u> <u>is</u> <u>not</u> <u>in</u>
<u>the medulla</u>; thus, if facial weakness is present there
must be dysfunction at the level of the pons or above.

When <u>descending</u> <u>sympathetic</u> <u>fibers</u> are involved,
an ipsilateral Horner's syndrome (ptosis, small pupil, and
facial anhidrosis) results.

<u>Cranial nerve nuclei</u>:

.<u>Twelfth</u> (hypoglossal): unilateral involvement of
nucleus causes fasciculations on that side; when the
tongue is protruded it deviates to the side of the
lesion.

.<u>Tenth</u> (vagus) and <u>ninth</u> (glossopharyngeal): these
innervate the laryngeal and pharyngeal musculature
and are motor and sensory nerves, respectively;
dysphagia is prominent when the vagus is involved.

PONS (Cranial Nerves 5 to 8)

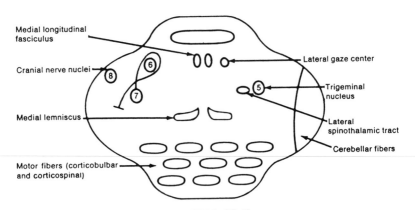

FIGURE 25.7

The fibers of the <u>seventh</u> (facial) <u>nerve</u> sweep around the sixth nerve (lateral rectus) before exiting from the pons. Thus, a lesion at this level may produce a sixth and seventh nerve paralysis on the same side.

Basic structure of the pons: medial involvement produces motor dysfunction and internuclear ophthalmoplegia or gaze palsy to the side of the lesion. Laterally there is sensory dysfunction.

<u>Vertical nystagmus</u> is a sign of brainstem dysfunction at the level of the pontomedullary junction (unless the patient is on barbiturates).

Eighth nerve nuclei include cochlear and vestibular components.

The <u>trigeminal nerve</u> exits from the middle of the pons and if <u>involved at this</u> level produces ipsilateral loss of the corneal reflex. In high pontine lesions pain and sensory loss are contralateral to the lesion in both face and extremities. Below the high pons, pain and temperature senses are lost ipsilaterally in the face and contralaterally in the limbs.

Lesions of the <u>medial longitudinal fasciculus</u> (MLF) result in an internuclear ophthalmoplegia. If the right MLF is involved there is difficulty with right eye adduction, as well as nystagmus in the abducting left eye when the patient looks to the left. This is the classic finding in demyelinating disease and can be seen in brainstem gliomas.

The most prominent disturbance in the midbrain generally involves the <u>third</u> <u>nerve</u> nucleus or exiting fibers, producing a dilated pupil and ophthalmoplegia.

Lesions affecting the area of the midbrain near the superior colliculus produce difficulty with upward gaze. A tumor pressing on the superior colliculus may present in this way (e.g., pinealoma).

Lesions of the red nucleus produce contralateral ataxia. The substantia nigra is located at this level and plays an important role in Parkinson's disease in the adult.

The <u>fourth</u> <u>nerve</u> nucleus is also located in the midbrain at a somewhat lower level and is seldom involved alone. (When it is involved alone, e.g., after head trauma, the clinical counterpart of fourth nerve dysfunction may be head tilt.)

Fibers from the optic tract concerned with the pupillary response synapse in the region of the third nerve nucleus.

MIDBRAIN (Cranial Nerves 3 to 4)

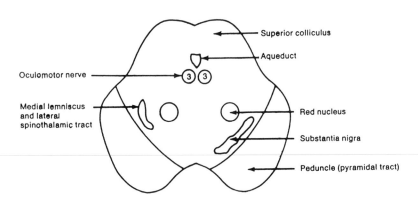

FIGURE 25.8

DERMATOME SENSORY CHART

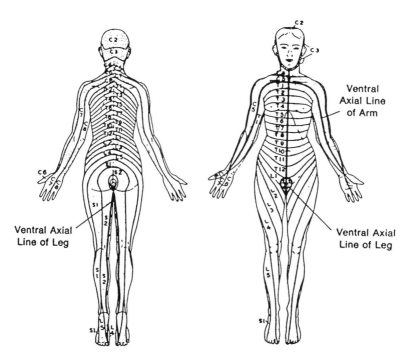

FIGURE 25.9

Left: dermatomes from the posterior view.
Right: dermatomes from the anterior view.
From Keegan JJ, Garrett FD: The segmental distribution of
the cutaneous nerves in the limbs of man. Anat Rec
102:409, 1948.
Reprinted by permission of the Wistar Institute Press,
Philadelphia, Pennsylvania.

Table 25.1 (Part 1)
CROSSINGS IN THE NERVOUS SYSTEM

Almost all major pathways in the nervous system
cross. Much of the understanding of neuroanatomy
relates to knowing where these tracts cross and thus
at which level the nervous system is involved.

Pathway	Function	Crosses	Interpretation
Pyramidal tract	Motor	Lower medulla	Lesion below crossing gives ipsilateral signs
Spino-thalamic tract	Pain and temperature (body)	On entry to spinal cord	Lesion is always contra-lateral to pain and temperature loss (except in face)
Spinal tract of fifth (V) nerve	Pain and temperature (face)	Midpons (runs through-out medulla)	If lesion is in medulla or lower pons, ipsilateral loss; above midpons, contralateral loss
Dorsal spinal columns	Position and vibration	Lower medulla	Lesion below crossing gives ipsilateral signs
Cere-bellar tracts	Coordina-tion of movement	Crosses twice (on entry to cerebellum and in midbrain)	Because of the "double crossing" lesions of cere-bellum or cere-bellar tracts usually produce signs and symptoms ipsilateral to lesion

Table 25.1 (Part 2)

CROSSINGS IN THE NERVOUS SYSTEM

Pathway	Function	Crosses	Interpretation
Gaze fibers	Coordinates lateral gaze	Midpons	See Figs. 6, 7 for interpretation
Cranial nerve fibers	Cranial nerves	Just above cranial nerve nuclei	Lesion is ipsilateral when cranial nerve nuclei are involved

214

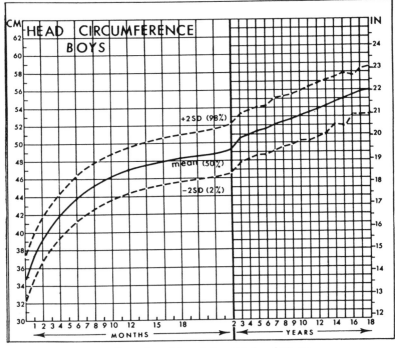

Composite graph for males from birth through 18 years.

FIGURE 25.10

From Nelhaus G: Head circumference from birth to eighteen years. Pediatrics 41:106, 1968; by permission.

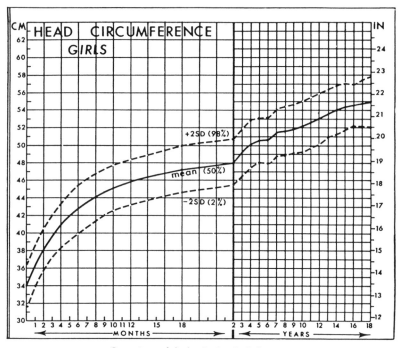

Composite graph for females from birth through 18 years.

FIGURE 25.11

216

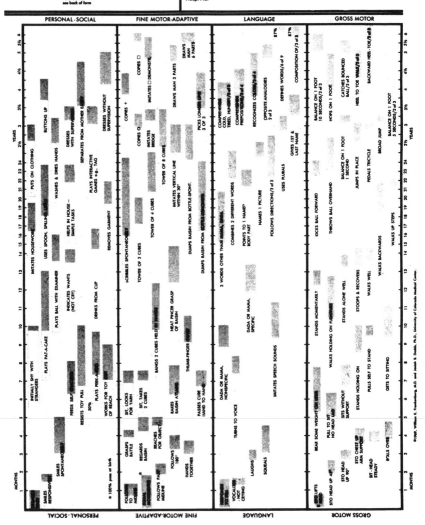

FIGURE 25.12

1. Try to get child to smile by smiling, talking or waving to him. Do not touch him.
2. When child is playing with toy, pull it away from him. Pass if he resists.
3. Child does not have to be able to tie shoes or button in the back.
4. Move yarn slowly in an arc from one side to the other, about 6" above child's face. Pass if eyes follow 90° to midline. (Past midline; 180°)
5. Pass if child grasps rattle when it is touched to the backs or tips of fingers.
6. Pass if child continues to look where yarn disappeared or tries to see where it went. Yarn should be dropped quickly from sight from tester's hand without arm movement.
7. Pass if child picks up raisin with any part of thumb and a finger.
8. Pass if child picks up raisin with the ends of thumb and index finger using an over hand approach.

9. Pass any enclosed form. Fail continuous round motions.
10. Which line is longer? (Not bigger.) Turn paper upside down and repeat. (3/3 or 5/6)
11. Pass any crossing lines.
12. Have child copy first. If failed, demonstrate

When giving items 9, 11 and 12, do not name the forms. Do not demonstrate 9 and 11.

13. When scoring, each pair (2 arms, 2 legs, etc.) counts as one part.
14. Point to picture and have child name it. (No credit is given for sounds only.)

15. Tell child to: Give block to Mommie; put block on table; put block on floor. Pass 2 of 3. (Do not help child by pointing, moving head or eyes.)
16. Ask child: What do you do when you are cold? ..hungry? ..tired? Pass 2 of 3.
17. Tell child to: Put block <u>on</u> table; <u>under</u> table; <u>in front</u> of chair, <u>behind</u> chair. Pass 3 of 4. (Do not help child by pointing, moving head or eyes.)
18. Ask child: If fire is hot, ice is ?; Mother is a woman, Dad is a ?; a horse is big, a mouse is ?. Pass 2 of 3.
19. Ask child: What is a ball? ..lake? ..desk? ..house? ..banana? ..curtain? ..ceiling? ..hedge? ..pavement? Pass if defined in terms of use, shape, what it is made of or general category (such as banana is fruit, not just yellow). Pass 6 of 9.
20. Ask child: What is a spoon made of? ..a shoe made of? ..a door made of? (No other objects may be substituted.) Pass 3 of 3.
21. When placed on stomach, child lifts chest off table with support of forearms and/or hands.
22. When child is on back, grasp his hands and pull him to sitting. Pass if head does not hang back.
23. Child may use wall or rail only, not person. May not crawl.
24. Child must throw ball overhand 3 feet to within arm's reach of tester.
25. Child must perform standing broad jump over width of test sheet. (8-1/2 inches)
26. Tell child to walk forward, ⊂⊃⊂⊃⊂⊃⊂⊃➤ heel within 1 inch of toe. Tester may demonstrate. Child must walk 4 consecutive steps, 2 out of 3 trials.
27. Bounce ball to child who should stand 3 feet away from tester. Child must catch ball with hands, not arms, 2 out of 3 trials.
28. Tell child to walk backward, ◄⊂⊃⊂⊃⊂⊃ toe within 1 inch of heel. Tester may demonstrate. Child must walk 4 consecutive steps, 2 out of 3 trials.

<u>DATE AND BEHAVIORAL OBSERVATIONS</u> (how child feels at time of test, relation to tester, attention span, verbal behavior, self-confidence, etc,):

FIGURE 25.12 (Continued)
By permission, W. Frankenburg.

Index

Page numbers in *italics* denote figures; those followed by "t" denote tables.